GET STRONGER, FEEL YOUNGER

GET STRONGER, FEEL YOUNGER

THE CARDIO- AND DIET-FREE PLAN TO
FIRM UP AND LOSE FAT

WAYNE WESTCOTT, PhD,
AND **GARY REINL**

RODALE

© 2007 by Wayne Westcott, PhD, and Gary Reinl

The recipes on pages 178 to 210: © 2003 and 2004 by Rodale Inc.

Rodale books may be purchased for business or promotional use or for special sales. For information, please write to: Special Markets Department, Rodale Inc., 733 Third Avenue, New York, NY 10017.

Printed in the United States of America

Rodale Inc. makes every effort to use acid-free ∞, recycled paper ♻.

Book design by Christina Gaugler

Interior photographs by Thomas MacDonald

Illustrations by Karen Kuchar

Library of Congress Cataloging-in-Publication Data

Westcott, Wayne L., date
    Get stronger, feel younger : the cardio- and diet-free plan to firm up and lose fat / Wayne Westcott and Gary Reinl.
        p.   cm.
    Includes index.
    ISBN-13 978–1–59486–689–0 hardcover
    ISBN-10 1–59486–689–9 hardcover
    1. Exercise.   2. Physical fitness.   3. Muscle strength.   I. Reinl, Gary R.   II. Title.
RA781.W417 2007
613.7'1—dc22   2007023661

Distributed to the trade by Holtzbrinck Publishers

2   4   6   8   10   9   7   5   3   1   hardcover

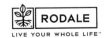

We inspire and enable people to improve their lives and the world around them

For more of our products visit **rodalestore.com** or call 1-800-848-4735

With great appreciation for their love, support, and assistance,
we gratefully dedicate this book to our wives,
Claudia Westcott and Susan Reinl.

CONTENTS

ACKNOWLEDGMENTS

We have been privileged to work with two outstanding Rodale editors, Courtney Conroy and Kevin Smith, and we are indebted to both of them for their excellent work. We are most grateful to Lois De La Haba for making this book possible, and to Buzz Truitt for his invaluable personal assistance and professional leadership with this project. We are particularly thankful to Jamie Robinson and Simone Strouble, our administrative associates, for their exceptionally fine work in preparing our manuscript.

Our extremely fit model, Olivia Chamberland, and our excellent design team of Marc Sirinsky, Christina Gaugler, Tom MacDonald, and Colleen Kobrick provided the superb exercise photos and book layout. We greatly appreciate all of the Rodale and *Prevention* team members, especially Michele Stanten, our fitness role model, Liz Vaccariello, Liz Perl, Nancy Hancock, and Francesca Minerva.

We also gratefully acknowledge Gregg Hammann, Tim Hawkins, Jim Brenner, Ron Arp, Bret Blount, and Kari Schunk at Nautilus for their expertise and for providing all of our exercise equipment. We also remember Arthur Jones and Dr. Ellington Darden for pioneering the strength-training techniques featured in our book.

We thank Ralph Yohe, Mary Hurley, Natalie Sheard, Mark Free, Rita La Rosa Loud, and Susan Stoddard at the South Shore YMCA for enabling us to conduct our extensive exercise studies. Finally, we could not conduct our research or write this text without God's grace and the support of our wonderful wives, Claudia Westcott and Susan Reinl. We thank you above all for your love and assistance.

FOREWORD

I f you want to get stronger and feel younger, pick up some dumbbells. As *Prevention*'s fitness director and an exercise instructor for the past 15 years, I have seen strength training, or lifting weights, turn back the clock and give many women just like you slimmer, firmer, healthier bodies—at any age. Now the Get Stronger, Feel Younger Plan, developed by Wayne Westcott, PhD, one of the top strength-training researchers in the country, gives you all the information you need to see fabulous results—whether you are picking up your first weights or have been lifting for years.

Strength training works because it targets one of the primary culprits of all those undesirable changes that occur as we age—muscle loss. Beginning as early as your twenties, you start to lose muscle—about $1/2$ pound a year. While that may not sound like much, when you consider all the roles that muscles play in your life, these little changes can have some big impacts.

Muscles fuel your body's metabolism—the amount of energy or number of calories your body uses every day to survive. The less muscle you have, the fewer calories your body burns, making it harder to lose weight or maintain a healthy weight. And muscle loss accelerates as you get older if you don't take action now.

Muscles make everyday activity easier. I'm sure you've seen a grandparent or other elderly person who's had trouble getting out of a chair or climbing stairs. The problem in many cases is a lack of muscle strength. Strong muscles will keep you moving with ease and most likely help you increase your everyday activity, which means you'll burn more calories. As you start to rebuild lost muscle, you may even feel so good that you'll be inspired to get back to activities you used to enjoy, such as cycling or dancing, or try something new like hiking, kickboxing, or tennis.

Muscles strengthen bones. As you get older, your bones start to weaken, increasing your risk of having a fracture. But the stronger your muscles are, the stronger your bones will be. Muscles pull on bones when you move, and the more powerful this action is, the more it will stimulate bones to get stronger. A strong skeletal system will also keep you standing taller and looking slimmer.

Muscles protect your joints. Back, knee, hip, and shoulder pain are common complaints as we age. By strengthening the muscles that surround and support these joints, you'll reduce your risk of injury, be more likely to remain pain-free, and feel younger.

Muscles give you a firmer, fitter-looking body. Because it's more compact than fat, muscle takes up less space. By losing fat through a healthy diet and exercise and building firm, calorie-burning muscle, you'll lose inches and be slipping into smaller sizes in no time.

And the benefits don't stop there. Strength training has also been shown to lower cholesterol, reduce blood pressure, decrease the risk of diabetes, improve moods, and raise confidence levels.

Now if you're like most women—myself included—you probably gravitate toward aerobic types of exercise, like walking. And that's good because cardio exercise is important for staying fit and slim . . . but it doesn't provide the muscle-building benefits that strength training does. If you really want to look and feel younger, you need to include weight lifting in your routine, and the Get Stronger, Feel Younger Plan can help.

For more than 35 years, Dr. Westcott, research director at the South Shore YMCA in Quincy, Massachusetts, and strength-training consultant to numerous organizations, has been studying the benefits of lifting weights in thousands of men, women, seniors, and kids—not athletes, but people just like you. So he understands the obstacles that can get in the way of maintaining a consistent routine. In this book, he's designed a variety of routines with simple yet effective moves. So you can pick the one that meets your needs—whether you're just adding strength training to your workouts or modifying a current program. And best of all, you can get started on your way to a leaner, firmer, stronger body in only 20 minutes a day, two or three times a week.

Michele Stanten
Fitness Director
Prevention® *Magazine*

INTRODUCTION

f you have too much fat, you are not alone. More than 75 percent of all Americans are "overfat." Even if you weigh the same 120 pounds at age 40 that you did in college, you most likely have 10 pounds more fat than you did when you were 20. How can that be if your body weight hasn't changed? Very simply, the average adult loses 5 to 7 pounds of muscle tissue every decade of life. So at age 40, your 120 pounds consists of 10 pounds less muscle and 10 pounds more fat than it should, which actually represents a 20-pound change in your body composition and physical appearance.

How did these undesirable changes occur? Moreover, how did they occur when you did not change your eating and exercise habits? If regular strength training is not a part of your weekly schedule, you lose approximately ½ pound of muscle tissue each year—even if you're a runner or an aerobic exerciser. Muscle is metabolically active tissue, which means that even at rest it uses calories to maintain itself. Accordingly, less muscle results in fewer calories burned on a daily basis. A 5- to 7-pound muscle loss leads to a 3 to 5 percent reduction in metabolic rate or calorie-burning capacity. And with a slower metabolism, more calories end up stored as fat.

How important is that? Really important! A slower metabolism is the primary cause of fat gain. It's that simple. Consider this common example.

Let's say that you have added 20 pounds of body weight over the past

10 years, even though your eating and exercise habits remained essentially the same. As you now know, those 20 extra pounds of body weight actually represent about 5 pounds less muscle and 25 pounds more fat. Assuming your initial resting metabolism was 1,000 calories per day, a 5 percent reduction in your calorie-burning capacity translates to 50 fewer calories (950 calories per day) needed by the end of the decade. Your daily calorie burn over the 10-year period would average about 25 fewer calories per day. This seemingly inconsequential reduction in your resting metabolism is actually responsible for your 25-pound fat gain. Just do the math—25 unused calories going into fat storage 365 days a year for 10 years is more than 90,000 accumulated calories. Because 1 pound of fat contains 3,500 calories, 90,000 calories represents just over 25 pounds of fat.

GET STRONGER, FEEL YOUNGER SUCCESS STORY

Roberta Norton, who represents many of our program participants, is a perfect case in point. Roberta's pre-strength-training life revolved around numerous diet plans, all of which failed to produce permanent weight loss. In fact, Roberta recounts that she would routinely begin a diet program on Monday and give up by Friday, experience feelings of failure over the weekend, and start a different diet program the following Monday. Roberta spent several years on the depressing diet roller coaster before deciding to try our strength-training approach for reducing fat. For fear of failing again, she didn't tell her family or friends that she had joined one of our YMCA strength-training classes. Within 2 weeks, she noticed firmer muscles and felt confident that she would lose fat, and she even promised herself that she would never diet again.

After the first 8 weeks, Roberta made major improvements in her appearance, adding 3 pounds of muscle and

It's important to understand that the 25 extra pounds of fat resulted from a relatively small reduction in resting metabolic rate. In this case, as in most others, the fat gain was not directly tied to eating too much or exercising too little. The real problem was muscle loss leading to metabolic slowdown and, in turn, fat gain.

The only successful solution is to rebuild the muscle tissue and recharge your metabolism. Fortunately, this is not hard to do. Most adults and seniors can rebuild 3 pounds of muscle in 10 weeks of sensible strength exercise. By sensible, we mean two or three training sessions a week, for just 20 to 30 minutes per session. Research reveals that training in this manner can increase your resting metabolic rate by more than 7 percent and your daily energy/calorie requirements by up to 15 percent. In addition, proper strength training

losing 10 pounds of fat. Within a few months, she reduced her body weight by almost 50 pounds, became extremely energetic, and engaged in a variety of physical activities she could not previously perform. After studying physical fitness and passing her national certification exam, Roberta became a certified personal trainer and has helped hundreds of other women (and men) attain lower body weight and better body composition through the Get Stronger, Feel Younger Plan of sensible strength exercise.

◄ Before

After ►

builds a strong, injury-resistant musculoskeletal system and provides a variety of health benefits, including reduced risk of diabetes, heart disease, osteoporosis, arthritis, depression, and several types of cancer.

What about dieting? You don't really need to follow a special diet—low-fat, low-carbohydrate, or otherwise—to deal with a 25-calorie-per-day metabolic deficit. What you need is muscle: the muscle you had a few years ago when you looked better, felt better, and functioned better. The muscle that gave you a higher metabolic rate and enabled you to eat normally without fat gain. Tragically, typical diet plans result in more muscle loss and metabolic rate reduction because approximately 25 percent of the weight you lose on a typical diet is actually muscle tissue.

We want you to realize that the dual problems of too little muscle and too much fat cannot be remedied by dieting alone. Even aerobic activity, such as walking, running, and cycling, as good as it is for cardiovascular fitness, will not restore your muscle tissue or raise your resting metabolic rate. The only way to replace your muscle and recharge your metabolism is through regular strength exercise. Essentially, you need to add muscle to lose fat. And that is what the Get Stronger, Feel Younger Plan is all about. As you become stronger, you'll look and feel younger because you'll reverse the three key factors that are involved in the aging process—muscle loss, metabolic slowdown, and fat gain. This plan rebuilds muscle, recharges metabolism, *and* reduces fat all at the same time.

The Get Stronger, Feel Younger Plan is not a calorie-restricted diet program that is practiced for a short period of time to produce temporary weight loss. Instead, this is a sensible, lifetime exercise plan that features basic and brief strength-training sessions that enable you to experience permanent fat loss and body composition benefits. This is the essential health and fitness program that helps you look, feel, and function better in as little as 10 weeks of exercise.

More than 3,000 research class participants have effectively applied the strength-training principles in this plan. Most had previously tried several popular diet programs, but few will do so again because they now know that the real solution for successful weight management and physical fitness is reducing their fat and remodeling their muscle. With the Get Stronger, Feel Younger Plan, you can achieve those very same goals.

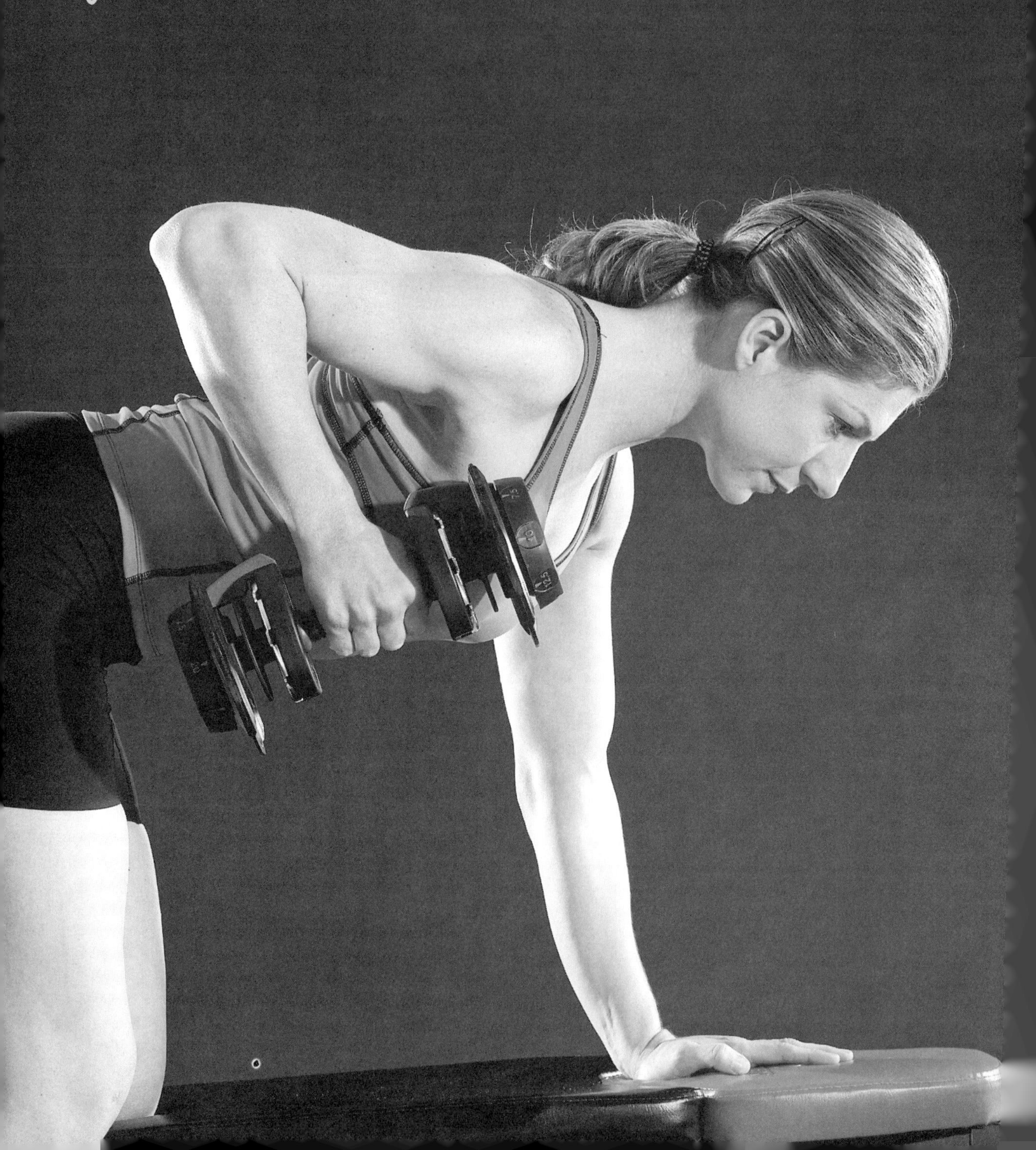

PART 1

TRANSFORM YOUR BODY

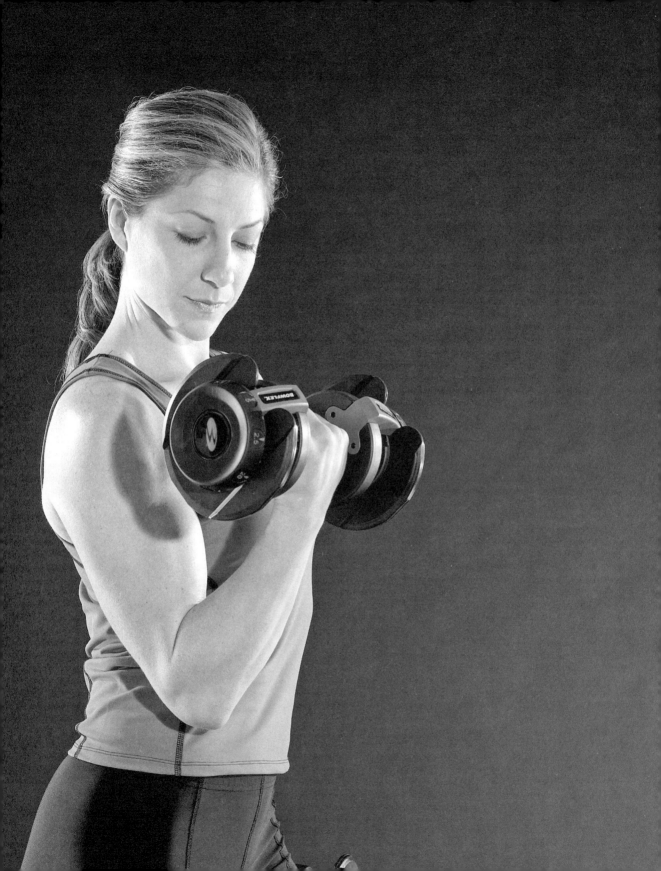

CHAPTER 1

THE ORIGINS
OF EXCESS FAT

D o you find yourself looking in the bathroom mirror and uncon-
sciously asking yourself, "How did I get so fat?" Sure, you're a little
less active than you used to be, which may explain how a *few* of the extra
inches got there. But what about the 30 additional pounds the bathroom scale
registers? You're not eating more food than you did in the past. In fact, you
may be dieting much of the time. There must be some other factor that is
making you look larger and feel softer. Indeed there is!

If you are an average adult who does not exercise regularly, you can lose
about 5 to 7 pounds of muscle every decade of life. If you are physically active,
you may lose a little less muscle tissue. If you diet frequently, you will undoubtedly lose significantly more muscle tissue. As we discussed earlier, muscle is a
very demanding tissue from a metabolic perspective, so consequently, less
muscle leads to a lower resting metabolism. Basically, 5 to 7 pounds less muscle
results in a 3 to 5 percent reduction in your resting metabolic rate. And

remember, this is a decade-by-decade reality that results in a cumulative slow-down in metabolism for most of us.

Less energy used by your muscular system means more calories stored in your fat cells, which is the underlying cause of the gradual fat gain experienced by 75 percent of Americans. Let's look at the sequence of events again, step by step.

Step 1. Lack of use causes you to lose muscle tissue at the rate of 5 to 7 pounds per decade throughout your adult years.

Step 2. Due to that reduction of very active muscle tissue, your metabolism slows down at a rate of 3 to 5 percent per decade as you age.

Step 3. Some of the calories that used to provide energy to your previously larger and stronger muscles are now stored in your fat cells, which causes an increase in your excess body fat and body weight.

GET STRONGER, FEEL YOUNGER SUCCESS STORY

Barbara Mendez found herself asking the question, "How did I get so fat?" Fortunately, she also asked her daughter, one of our best strength-training instructors, what she could do to change her condition. Here is what Barbara had to say after experiencing our Get Stronger, Feel Younger Plan for permanent fat loss.

"I wanted to join a program I could commit to; this program was a commitment of three times per week. The exercises were realistic and time efficient, making it an enjoyable experience. The diet was easy to follow. It's well balanced and offers a variety of foods. I never felt deprived as I have on other diets. My body shape changed very quickly. My clothes fit better almost immediately. My posture is even better. I stand taller now. My thighs are smoother; that's for sure. There were times I could see little lumps and bumps through my

Obviously, you can determine how much weight you've gained by stepping on the bathroom scale. However, the scale only provides you with a fraction of your overall weight-gain picture. The number looking up at you represents your net change in body weight. But that typically represents only half of the real problem. If you take a careful look at Figure 1 on page 6, you'll see that the average American woman adds about 10 pounds per decade in total body weight, as indicated by the bathroom scale. However, you will also see that she actually loses 5 pounds of muscle and gains roughly 15 pounds of fat on a decade-by-decade basis. Five pounds less muscle combined with 15 pounds more fat equals a 20-pound change in the average woman's body composition, or muscle-to-fat ratio. In other words, what the scale might indicate to you as a simple 10-pound problem (10 pounds more body weight) is actually a complex 20-pound problem (15 pounds more fat and 5 pounds less muscle).

Notice that by age 50, the average American woman has added 30 pounds

clothes. Now they've disappeared! I plan to continue to follow this program. I tell everyone, it's a way of life!"

Barbara actually lost 16 pounds of unsightly fat and replaced them with 3 pounds of attractive muscle during her 2-month strength-training program. That is, she reduced her body weight by 13 pounds, but she improved her body composition and personal appearance by 19 pounds. This represents a remarkable change rate of almost 2.5 pounds per week. Through her exercise efforts and dietary modifications, Barbara reduced her percent body fat by six points and her hip measurement by almost 3 inches. She no longer asks, "How did I get so fat?" because she now knows firsthand how sensible strength exercise replaces muscle and reduces fat for a better figure in a brief training period.

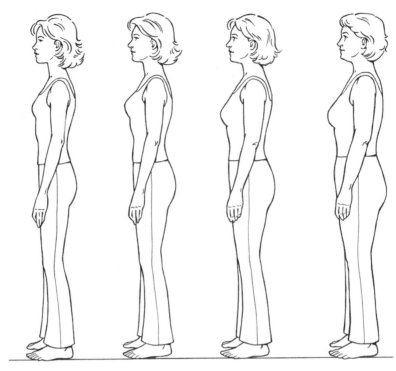

Age	20	30	40	50
Body weight (lb)	126	136	146	156
Muscle (lb)	45	40	35	30
Fat (lb)	29	44	59	74
Percent fat	23	32	40	47

Figure 1. Decade-by-decade changes in body weight and body composition in the average American woman.

of body weight. In actuality, she has changed her body composition by 60 pounds (45 pounds more fat and 15 pounds less muscle), and she is almost half (47 percent) fat. This amount of body fat is extremely unhealthy and significantly increases the risk of numerous degenerative diseases such as diabetes, stroke, heart problems, osteoporosis, arthritis, back pain, and some types of cancer. Not to be outdone, the average American man loses *even more* muscle and adds even more fat throughout his adult life. On average, men lose about

7 pounds of muscle and gain about 17 pounds of fat on a decade-by-decade basis.

It is possible to have more fat than necessary and still be relatively fit if you do enough exercise to keep your muscles firm and strong. Many professional athletes fall into this category. However, if you do not maintain a desirable level of muscular fitness, you will look softer and and feel larger on account of too much fat on top of too little muscle. In essence, having an underlying muscle foundation that is too thin and an overlying fat layer that is too thick will result in a roly-poly appearance. When this slow but insidious process progresses too far, the unsupported fat may form little lumps and bumps you know as cellulite.

Of course, eating more calories than you need to makes this unhealthy situation even worse by increasing the rate of fat storage, but you undoubtedly know that. What you need to remember is that popular reduced-calorie diets are even more damaging to your metabolism and almost always result in greater fat gain than fat loss over time. Although a few people appear to benefit from dieting, research reveals that 95 percent of *successful* dieters have more fat 1 year after their diet than before they began dieting. These are not good odds, and the potential health consequences are even worse. You'll learn more about the detrimental effects of diets in Chapter 2.

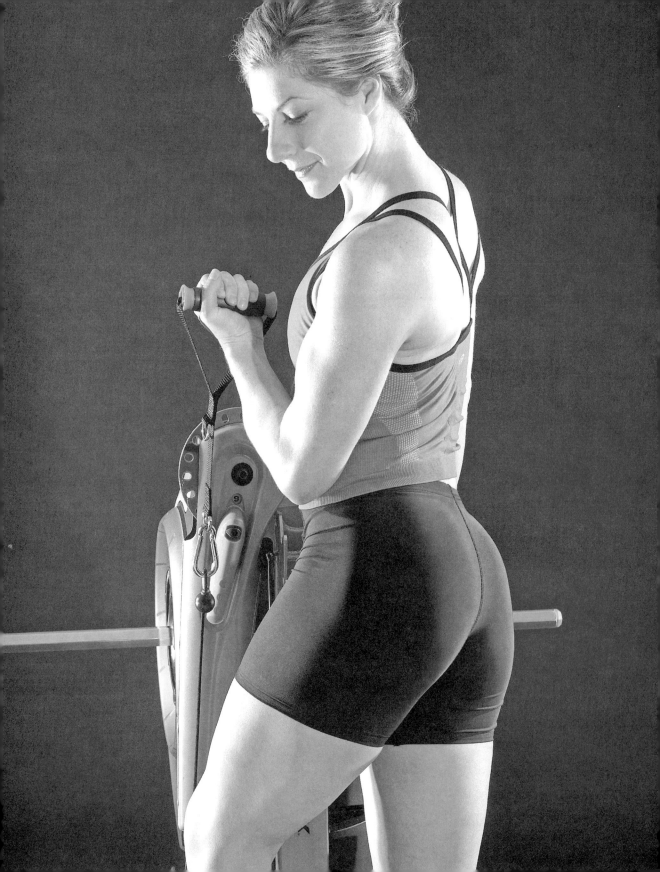

WHY DON'T DIET PLANS WORK?

Today, one of every two American adults is following some form of reduced-calorie diet plan. From a monetary perspective, dieters in the United States spend well over $45 billion annually on various reduced-calorie diet programs. If these diet plans were even moderately successful, we would be a nation of lean people. Obviously, this is not the case. In fact, U.S. government figures show that about 65 percent of adults are overweight, while an Ohio University study shows that fully 75 percent of American adults are over*fat*. So, on average, 7 out of every 10 men and women need to lose excess fat.

Unfortunately, research reveals that dieting alone is not an effective means for attaining permanent weight loss. One study showed that 50 percent of those who start a diet program drop out before they achieve their desired body weight. Another study found that 95 percent of those who succeed on their diet program regain all the weight they lost within 1 year.

In a very real sense, dieting is like knocking yourself out temporarily so that you don't feel the pain of a headache. When you eventually regain consciousness, however, the headache is much worse than before you "treated" it. Here's why the comparison is pretty close to the mark. When you follow a reduced-calorie diet plan (pick any popular diet program you want), you place yourself in an energy-deficit situation. Basically, you are not eating enough food to supply your daily energy requirements. In order to live, let alone exercise, you must make up for the imposed energy deficit by utilizing tissue sources like the fat and muscle within your body to supply the energy you need.

The primary source of energy in the body is fat stored in your fat cells. After that, there is glycogen, which is a form of sugar stored in your liver and muscle tissues. Unfortunately, it takes longer for your body to mobilize these energy sources than is necessary to make up for the energy deficit caused by most reduced-calorie diet programs. As a result, your body breaks down muscle tissue to get the additional energy you need to make up the difference.

Why doesn't reduced-calorie dieting work?

Obviously, what makes reduced-calorie dieting so popular is the relatively rapid loss of body weight it causes. While most of that weight loss comes from fat, up to 25 percent of the weight loss comes from muscle. That's right, reduced-calorie diets almost always result in muscle loss, which reduces your resting metabolic rate and makes it almost impossible to keep the weight off.

Let's look at some numbers. Let's say you previously weighed 180 pounds, and you diligently dieted your weight down to 140 pounds. You lost 40 pounds. Perhaps 30 of those pounds came from fat (good) and perhaps 10 of those pounds came from muscle (bad). At rest, 10 pounds of muscle consumes a lot of calories every day to maintain itself, unlike fat. This factor, coupled with the metabolic slowdown that always accompanies rapid weight loss, may reduce your resting metabolic rate by as much as 350 calories per day.

Normally, most people won't starve themselves indefinitely and they eventually return to their normal eating patterns. When you do, the same number of daily calories that you previously needed to maintain your body weight may now be 350 calories more than your now-reduced resting metabolism can accommodate. And guess what? These 350 extra calories are sent into your body's fat-storage areas. Other things being equal, you regain a pound of fat every 10 days (350 calories per day × 10 days = 3,500 calories = 1 pound of fat). In 1 year, you will have added 36 pounds of fat (see the table below). You will have exceeded by 6 pounds the 30 pounds of fat that you lost on the diet program. And if that isn't bad enough, you will look fatter and less fit than before your diet because you sacrificed several pounds of firm muscle through the dieting process.

EXAMPLE OF TYPICAL DIETING RESPONSES

	BEFORE DIET	AFTER DIET	1 YEAR AFTER DIET	REAL CHANGE
BODY WEIGHT	180 lb	140 lb	180 lb	Same
FAT WEIGHT	60 lb	30 lb	66 lb	+6 lb fat
LEAN WEIGHT (MUSCLE, BONE, ETC.)	120 lb	110 lb	114 lb	−6 lb muscle
BODY FAT PERCENTAGE	33%	21%	37%	+4% body fat

Think about this logically. One year after *succeeding* on a reduced-calorie diet program, 95 percent of all dieters weigh as much as they did before dieting, but they now have more fat and less muscle. Sounds pathetic, right? All the time, money, and effort spent on dieting is short-circuited by muscle loss and metabolic slowdown, leading rather quickly to a fatter body that looks worse, feels worse, and functions less efficiently than it did before you started starving yourself.

Quite simply, dieting doesn't work because it results in muscle loss and metabolic reduction that negatively impact your health and fitness—not to mention your personal appearance and physical function. Eventually, your body rebounds to a higher body weight and a poorer body composition. Basically, dieting is like simultaneously filling your pickup truck with bricks (fat gain) and changing your engine from eight cylinders to four cylinders (muscle loss). Such a situation will put unnecessary stress on your truck. Similarly, dieting will stress your body and cause a host of problems beyond just an unhealthy, inefficient body composition.

If you are accustomed to constantly dieting, the thought of discontinuing a strict diet plan can seem counterintuitive to your goals, but hear us out. By combining a sensible diet plan that includes *all* of the essential food groups (with an emphasis on a variety of healthful vegetables, fruits, and grains) with regular strength training, you can achieve the very same goals. The U.S.

Department of Agriculture Food Guide Pyramid, MyPyramid, represents a sound and balanced nutrition program that is widely accepted by dietitians, doctors, and health professionals alike (see Chapter 10 for details). To reduce your food consumption, you may choose a 2,800-, 2,200-, or 1,600-calorie-per-day diet plan that cuts equally across all of the food categories without eliminating any essential nutrients.

Whether you decide to diet independently or join a support group such as Weight Watchers or TOPS, be sure to perform regular strength exercise to maintain your muscle tissue and metabolic rate. An appropriate nutrition plan coupled with regular strength training may work as well for you as it did for Kathy Tully.

If you, like Kathy, have experienced little success with diet plans, it is most likely not your fault. Although diet plans are widely promoted as the best means for losing weight, their value is temporary at best. Diet plans typically cause more problems than they solve. As we mentioned earlier, the inevitable result of popular reduced-calorie diet plans is muscle loss and metabolic slowdown that make it nearly impossible to avoid regaining all of the fat that you previously lost.

As you have probably noticed, dieting is seldom a simple process and most certainly not an enjoyable one. But we have good news for you! The Get Stronger, Feel Younger Plan is simple to understand and implement. It is efficient from a time perspective. It's effective for both decreasing your body weight and improving your body composition, or muscle-to-fat ratio, because it concurrently reduces fat, replaces muscle, and recharges your metabolism. As you read the next chapter, you should be pleasantly surprised to learn how building your muscles—not dieting—is the ideal approach for losing your excess fat.

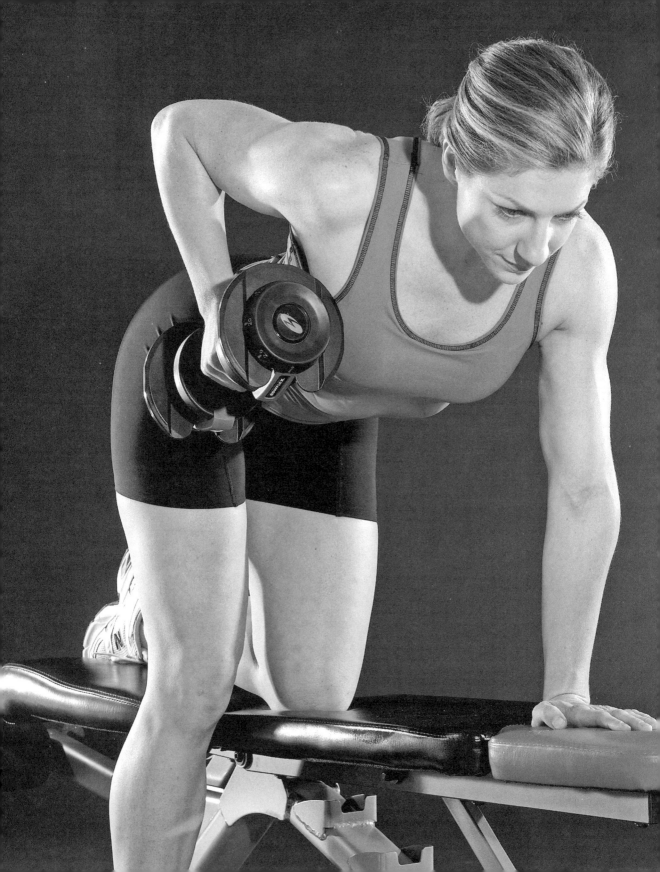

CHAPTER 3

HOW DO STRONG MUSCLES REDUCE FAT?

M ost of us have been led to believe that the best way to lose body weight is through a reduced-calorie diet plan that decreases the number of calories we consume. Some of us, who have more enthusiasm for exercise, have learned that regular aerobic activity can also contribute to weight loss by increasing the number of calories we burn. However, few of us have heard that remodeling muscle is by far the most effective means for achieving permanent fat loss. That's right, building muscle through safe and sensible strength training essentially guarantees fat loss, as you will see in this chapter.

It's crucial to remember that the two basic physiological problems associated with the aging process are:

- Muscle loss of about 5 to 7 pounds per decade
- Fat gain of about 15 to 17 pounds per decade

Recall that less muscle leads to a lower resting metabolic rate that is largely responsible for the increase in fat weight. Because reduced-calorie diets almost always result in additional muscle loss, dieting alone is likely to do more harm than good in the long run.

YOUR MUSCLES ON THE RUN . . . AND IN THE WEIGHT ROOM

Aerobic activity is, of course, a better approach to weight loss than dieting because it does not typically cause muscle loss. However, you have to do relatively large amounts of aerobic activity to lose just 1 pound of fat. That means about 35 miles of running to lose just 1 pound! Endurance exercise uses the highly efficient aerobic system of energy production. Basically, walking, running, cycling, and similar endurance exercises burn calories while they are being performed. However, after this type of workout, you quickly return to your resting level of energy expenditure, where you are no longer burning calories at a high rate. Additionally, endurance exercise does not build muscle, so your resting metabolic rate remains essentially the same.

Strength training builds muscle tissue (replacing what was lost through inactivity or never developed in the first place) and increases your resting metabolic rate, allowing you to burn more calories even when you are not working out. Muscle-building exercise uses the highly inefficient anaerobic system of energy production. This anaerobic energy system functions without oxygen and requires approximately 20 times as much glucose as the aerobic energy system to produce the same amount of energy. These anaerobic energy sources must be replenished aerobically after the training period. Research from Southeastern Louisiana University revealed that during the hour following a 20-minute circuit strength-training session, the participants burned 25 percent as many calories during their postworkout metabolic slowdown as they did during the actual exercise period. Other research from Colorado State University has shown elevated resting metabolic rates more than 12 hours after completion of a strenuous strength-training session. So muscle-building exercise actually has a double effect on energy utilization, both during and after the workout.

For example, you may burn about 8 calories per minute during a circuit of short-rest strength-building exercise. So, a 30-minute circuit-training session of muscle-building exercise will require about 240 calories of energy utilization. During the hour following your strength-training workout, you may burn 60 additional calories to replenish the anaerobic energy supplies used to perform the exercises. Therefore, the actual energy cost of the 30-minute circuit training session is 300 calories, which is 50 percent more calories than you would typically use for a 30-minute walk (6.5 calories per minute or 200 total calories).

But the benefits of brief and basic muscle-building sessions for reducing body fat are even more impressive. In addition to burning calories during and after your workouts, as you increase your muscle tissue, you will burn more calories all day long. Our studies with thousands of men and women who have participated in our strength-training research classes show an average muscle gain of 3 pounds in less than 3 months (about 1 pound per month). According to studies conducted at Tufts University, the University of Maryland, and the University of Alabama, the same strength-training program that builds 3 pounds of muscle produces a 6 to 7 percent increase in resting metabolic rate.

A GET STRONGER, FEEL YOUNGER YOU?

Let's say that your pretraining resting metabolism was 1,600 calories a day. After about 3 months of muscle-building exercise, you have developed 3 more pounds of muscle and conditioned all of your major muscle groups. The combination of more muscle and more active tissue raises your resting metabolic rate by 6.5 percent, which translates to about 104 extra calories burned every day. Just by maintaining the resting energy needs of your strength-trained muscle tissue, you will burn 728 additional calories every week or about 3,000 more calories every month (which equals almost 11 pounds of fat loss in a year). The added bonus: Your new resting metabolism is now more than 1,700 calories a day!

Now you know that muscle-building exercise has a triple effect when it comes to reducing body fat. First, you burn extra calories when you perform muscle-building exercise. Second, you burn extra calories for several hours following your strength-training workout to replenish energy sources. Third, you burn extra calories all day long (including while you sleep) due to greater metabolic activity in conditioned muscle tissue. As you can see, strengthening your muscles is a highly effective means for reducing excess fat.

Consider the following example. Let's say you begin your muscle-building exercise program with a body weight of 172 pounds and a fat reading of 32 percent. Essentially, you have 55 pounds of fat weight and 117 pounds of muscle or lean weight. After 12 weeks of basic and brief strength training (12 exercise sets for the major muscle groups, 3 days a week), you add 3 pounds of lean (muscle) weight, and you lose 4 pounds of fat weight. This accounts for a 7-pound improvement in your body composition, an increase in resting metabolic rate of about 7 percent, and a total daily energy expenditure increase of 15 percent (about 300 calories a day). You may assume this is a hypothetical situation that is too good to be true, but it is actually the average result experienced by 12 senior men and women in the Tufts University study referred to earlier in this chapter. Keep in mind that the Tufts researchers fed the study participants more food each week in order to maintain their original body weight. If participants had continued to eat the same number of daily calories, their 300-calorie-per-day increase in energy expenditure could have led to a 30-pound fat loss over the course of a year. Considering that these study subjects were not trying to reduce their body weight, just think how well a similar strength-training program can work for you. It is really hard to beat a basic and brief program of sensible muscle-building exercise for safely, effectively, and efficiently improving your body composition and physical appearance.

Replacing the muscle you've lost during an inactive aging process through strength training is like replacing a four-cylinder automobile engine with an eight-cylinder: By replacing a smaller engine (a body with lost muscle) with a bigger engine (a body with newly gained muscle), you'll get more power and burn more calories (both when you are active and when you are inactive). Going a step further, many adults in our exceptionally sedentary society have never developed a desirable level of muscular strength in the first place, so they desperately need to do some muscle-building activity. Muscles are the engines of the body, and as the analogy indicates, better muscular engines lead to better body composition, personal appearance, and physical function.

If you are worried about building too much muscle, rest assured that this is most unlikely. As fitness professionals, we have been trying to build big muscles for 40 years. In reality, very few men, and even fewer women, possess the genetic potential to develop large muscles. So don't be concerned that you will become a muscle-bound behemoth by strength training a few days a week. You are simply trying to replace the muscle tissue that you may have lost due to inactivity over the past 10 to 20 years and/or that you never developed in the first place. We think you will be very pleased with your well-conditioned muscles that make you look firm and fit and enable you to feel and function so much better.

LOOKING BACK . . . HINDSIGHT IS 20/20

It is tempting to say that muscles eat fat and that strong muscles eat more fat. In a sense this is true, because it accurately portrays the eventual outcome. However, the intermediate process involves the use of two energy sources, namely stored glycogen and stored fat. Other things being equal, all of the extra calories used by your muscles during the workout, after the workout, and throughout the day are ultimately resupplied from your fat stores, which reduces your overall body fat accordingly. It is really amazing to learn how large a role your muscles play in the fat-loss process!

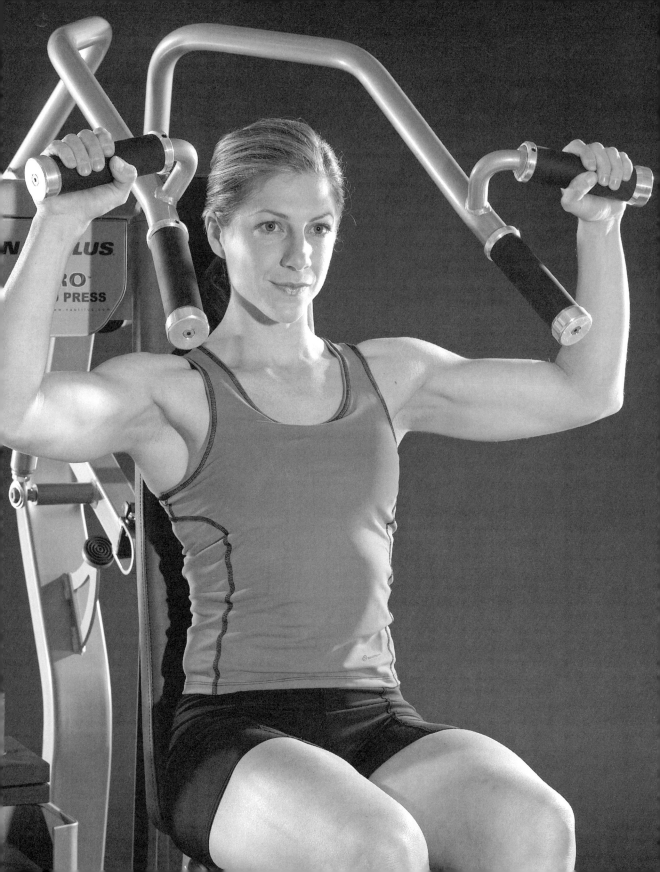

CHAPTER 4

HOW DO I DEVELOP STRONG MUSCLES?

You perceive muscle-building exercise as something you see on television during the Olympic Games when very strong (and very large) men and women lift tremendously heavy weights over their heads as powerfully as possible. This is actually the sport of weight lifting, which has little relationship to the type of strength training you will be doing on the Get Stronger, Feel Younger Plan. You may also have seen sports segments where very muscular men and women perform various poses in physique contests. These are professional bodybuilders whose extensive and intense exercise programs also have little similarity to the basic and brief strength-training programs you will be following. While you may have previously considered strength training to be the exclusive domain of football players and other larger-than-life athletes, this assumption bears little truth. About half of the teams in the National Football League train in a manner comparable to our recommended muscle-building protocols. Oh yes, the football players are larger and stronger with different training objectives, but the essential aspects of their muscle-building programs are quite similar to ours. Let's take a look at a simple, sensible, and successful strategy for developing strong muscles in a safe, effective, and time-efficient manner.

TRAINING FREQUENCY

Before you commit to a muscle-building exercise program, you need to know how often you will be exercising. We have conducted several studies on the effects of different strength-training techniques, and the results have been pleasantly surprising from a practical perspective. One of our largest studies involved more than 1,200 new exercisers who performed exactly the same weight workout either 1, 2, or 3 days each week for a 2-month training program. We carefully assessed the participants' changes in body composition over the training period. As presented in the table below, those who trained 3 days a week made the greatest body composition improvement, adding 2.5 pounds of muscle and losing 4.6 pounds of fat. Participants who trained 2 days a week experienced more than 85 percent as much body composition improvement, adding 2.2 pounds of muscle and losing 4.0 pounds of fat. Those who trained only 1 day a week made almost 70 percent as much body composition improvement, adding 1.7 pounds of muscle and losing 3.0 pounds of fat.

8-WEEK CHANGES IN BODY COMPOSITION

	3 DAYS/WEEK	2 DAYS/WEEK	1 DAY/WEEK
MUSCLE GAIN	2.5 lb	2.2 lb	1.7 lb
FAT LOSS	4.6 lb	4.0 lb	3.0 lb

In our follow-up study, more than 1,600 participants performed the same strength workouts either twice a week or 3 days a week for a period of 10 weeks. In this longer study, both training frequencies produced identical increases in lean (muscle) weight. The subjects who exercised on Tuesdays and Thursdays gained 3.1 pounds of muscle, and those who exercised on Mondays, Wednesdays, and Fridays also gained 3.1 pounds of muscle. Apparently, when training for more than 10 weeks, two or three weight workouts a week are equally beneficial for rebuilding your muscles. The fact that different training frequencies proved effective for improving body composition allows some freedom in your schedule, depending on what you are comfortable doing and how much time you have. For the best results, you should strength train 2 or 3 nonconsecutive days a week, but even one good exercise session a week is sufficient. Our bet is that you can find a way to fit at least one muscle-building workout into your weekly schedule.

TRAINING TIME

There are several exercise considerations that will affect the length of your strength-training session. At the top of this list is the number of exercises that you perform during your individual workout. We advise performing 8 to 12 different exercises per session as a beginner, and no more than 12 to 16 exercises per session as an advanced trainee. Assuming that you perform one set of each exercise in approximately 1 minute and that you take about a minute of rest between exercises, an eight-station workout should require about 15 minutes while a 12-station workout should require about 20 minutes, and a 16-station workout should require approximately 30 minutes. As you can see, our suggested strength-training programs are relatively brief, requiring only 15 to 30 minutes per session, depending on the number of exercises you perform.

Obviously, you will increase your training time if you choose to do more than one set of each exercise. For example, if you do two sets of eight exercises, it will increase your workout time from 15 minutes to almost 40 minutes (1 minute for each of 16 exercise sets, 2 minutes between successive sets of the same exercise, and 1 minute between exercises). Fortunately, most research regarding the number of sets per exercise indicates that one properly executed set is as effective as multiple sets. Using the Get Stronger, Feel Younger Plan, you should properly perform one set of each exercise to minimize training time, reduce your risk of overtraining injuries, and accommodate your schedule. Even the busiest individuals can find time for two weekly 15-minute muscle-building workouts.

TRAINING SETS

As you read above, we prefer single-set strength training because it is both effective and time efficient. From a physiological perspective, a psychological perspective, and a practical perspective, single-set strength training makes good sense. However, you may wonder if single-set training protocols produce as much strength as multiple-set training protocols. Our research, as well as numerous other studies on this topic, has shown no significant differences between training with one, two, or three sets of strength exercises.

Exercise intensity is the key to muscle development, while time is often a prohibitive factor for most exercisers. That's why this program has you perform one properly executed set of each strength exercise to achieve optimum muscle development. This training protocol has worked extremely well for our program participants, and we are confident it will do the same for you.

8-WEEK CHANGES IN MUSCLE STRENGTH
(MEASURED BY ADDITIONAL REPETITIONS)

	3 SETS/EXERCISE	2 SETS/EXERCISE	1 SET/EXERCISE
STRENGTH IMPROVEMENT	+5 repetitions	+4 repetitions	+4 repetitions

Single-set strength training is essentially as effective as multiple-set strength training, and because it takes so much less workout time, we suggest that you start training with one set of each exercise. Even our advanced high-intensity strength-training programs are based on single-set training protocols. In fact, almost half of the teams in the National Football League employ single-set, high-intensity strength-training protocols in their conditioning programs. If one good exercise set works for them, think how well it will work for you.

TRAINING REPETITIONS AND RESISTANCE

Just as the cell is the basic building block of the body, the repetition is the basic building block of your muscle-building program. Nothing is more critical to successful muscle building than proper execution of your exercise repetitions. How you perform repetitions and how many repetitions you perform are closely related aspects of your exercise program. So let's first take a look at the number of repetitions you should complete during each exercise set.

Our basic assumption is that you perform each set of strength exercise to the point of temporary muscle fatigue. That is, you do as many repetitions as you can complete with proper form. Obviously, there is a strong correlation between the amount of resistance you use and the number of repetitions you can perform. In fact, the resistance-repetition relationships presented in the following table are characteristic for most men and women.

RESISTANCE-REPETITION RELATIONSHIPS

MAXIMUM RESISTANCE (%)	100	95	90	85	80	75	70	65	60
AVERAGE REPETITIONS	1	2	4	6	8	10	12	14	16

Given the normal resistance-repetition relationships, we find that most adults experience excellent results training within the middle range of repetitions (8 to 12 reps), which corresponds to the middle range of resistance (70 to 80 percent of maximum). Although other repetitions protocols are also productive, performing 8 to 12 repetitions to muscle fatigue has proven to be highly effective both physiologically and psychologically. This is because 8 to 12 properly performed repetitions require about 50 to 70 seconds for completion, which is not too short or too long, and use about 70 to 80 percent of maximum resistance, which is not too light or too heavy.

While you may be inclined to think that performing more repetitions is beneficial for burning more calories, the extra energy expenditure from a few additional repetitions is actually quite small. Remember that the main purpose of your strength training is to build muscle, which requires relatively heavy resistance and reasonably high effort. Doing 8 to 12 repetitions per exercise set has produced excellent results in thousands of our research program participants. On the Get Stronger, Feel Younger Plan, you should begin your strength training with 8 to 12 repetitions per set. You can always modify your program later.

TRAINING PROGRESSION

Gaining muscle strength is an exciting process that requires progressive increases in your exercise resistance. That is, you should regularly add more resistance to stimulate greater muscle development. Although some trainers advocate increasing the resistance weekly, muscles do not necessarily adapt to stress in an optimum manner every 7 days. Some muscle groups respond faster than others, and because people differ physiologically, we recommend a simple progression procedure based on the number of repetitions you can presently perform. Basically, you should keep training with the same amount of weight until you can complete at least 12 good repetitions. Once you complete 12 repetitions with proper form twice in a row, you can increase the resistance by about 5 percent for your next workout. This will typically reduce the number of repetitions you can perform by two or three, but it will keep you in the preferred training range of 8 to 12 repetitions. This way, you can properly target individual muscle groups, progressing more quickly with faster-responding muscles, such as the larger muscles of the legs, while progressing more slowly with slower-responding muscles, like the smaller muscles in the arms.

For example, if you are presently performing 10 leg extensions with 50 pounds, stay with this resistance until you can complete 12 repetitions in proper form for two workouts in succession. When you can complete this, increase the resistance by 5 percent to about 52.5 pounds. Keep training with this resistance until you can complete 12 good repetitions two sessions in a row, then add another 5 percent to about 55 pounds. This double-progressive training, first increasing repetitions and then adding resistance, is both reasonable and effective. It requires a little patience, but it prevents you from doing too much too soon and ensures a muscle-matched improvement that is hard to beat.

TRAINING SPEED

When it comes to proper training technique, nothing is more misunderstood than repetition speed. Many people mistakenly believe that faster movements are more productive movements, but this is a misconception. Fast repetitions place more emphasis on momentum and less emphasis on muscle tension. Specifically, fast movements require very high muscle effort to initiate the repetition, but very little muscle effort throughout the remainder of the repetition. This type of training is characterized by increased injury risk and decreased muscle development, both of which are undesirable.

To minimize your risk of injury while maximizing muscle development, simply slow your repetition speed. While no one has identified the perfect speed for performing muscle-building exercises, the key is to control the resistance throughout each lifting and lowering movement. This means that you can stop the repetition at any point in the range of motion, because you are using controlled muscle effort rather than uncontrolled momentum.

Generally speaking, the lifting phase of most exercises should take about 2 seconds, with longer-range movements taking more time to complete. Simply count "one thousand one, one thousand two" (or more for longer movements) as you perform the lifting action. You can produce approximately 40 percent more strength during muscle-lengthening actions than during muscle-shortening actions. That is, you can lower about 40 percent more resistance than you can lift. For this reason, we recommend performing your lowering movements about twice as slow as your lifting movements. As a rule, the lowering phase of most exercises should take about 4 seconds, with longer-range movements taking more time to complete. When you train in this manner (about 2 seconds for lifting actions and about 4 seconds for lowering actions), you challenge the target muscles during both phases of each exercise repetition, thereby attaining better results.

You don't need to use a stopwatch to time your repetitions. After performing several exercises at about 6 seconds per repetition each (2 seconds lifting and 4 seconds lowering), you should find this training procedure comfortable, challenging, and almost second nature. Just remember that longer exercise movements will take more than 6 seconds per repetition. If you are ever in doubt about your repetition speed, we suggest that you try moving slower rather than faster because this almost always improves the training response.

TRAINING RANGE

Another important component of proper exercise technique is your exercise range of movement. Rotary movement exercises, such as leg curls and arm curls, should normally be performed through a full range of joint movement bounded by end positions of full flexion and full extension. Linear movement exercises, such as leg presses and chest presses, should normally be performed through a comfortable range of joint motion. Of course, you should never move into an exercise position that causes joint discomfort.

Basically, full-range exercise movements ensure full-range strength gains and maximum muscle development, which are important training objectives.

On the other hand, abbreviated exercise movements can lead to unbalanced muscles as well as less muscle development and should be avoided. When you perform your exercises with full movement range and controlled movement speed, you maximize the muscle-building benefits of your program. Remember that your main objective is to build stronger muscles to lose more fat.

TRAINING POSTURE AND EXERCISE BREATHING

Proper posture is important while performing your strength-training exercises in order to decrease the risk of injury and to increase the muscle-building benefits. You should always stand or sit erect when executing your exercise repetitions. Generally speaking, you should maintain your spine in a neutral position throughout most exercises, except during lower back extensions and trunk flexions. Specifically, you should avoid slouching forward, arching backward, or bending sideward, as well as throwing your head forward, backward, or to either side when you are performing your repetitions. Try to be comfortably tall (stand tall, sit tall) during strength-training exercises.

Proper breathing technique involves continuous air exchange on every repetition of every exercise. Never hold your breath when you are strength training because this can cause undesirable increases in blood pressure. You should exhale during each lifting movement and inhale throughout each lowering movement (breathing through your nose and mouth). Practice breathing out during the lifting actions and breathing in during the lowering actions until this pattern becomes automatic. Breathing in this manner is beneficial both physiologically and psychologically and ensures constant air flow throughout each exercise.

TRAINING EXERCISES

Your main objective is to exercise all of your major muscle groups in a balanced and comprehensive manner. These include the larger muscles of the legs, midsection, and upper body, as well as the smaller muscles of the arms and neck.

You can effectively train your major muscles in two ways. One, you can perform single-joint exercises that target a single muscle group, such as the quadriceps or deltoids. These exercises are always performed with rotary (curved) movements, such as leg extensions or lateral raises. Two, you can perform multiple-joint exercises that concurrently involve two or more major muscle groups, such as the quadriceps, hamstrings, and gluteals together, or the deltoids and triceps together. These exercises are always performed with linear (straight) movements, such as leg presses or shoulder presses.

Chapter 5 presents our recommended strength-training exercises for building a strong, fit, and functional musculoskeletal system. However, the following table provides a basic exercise format for a comprehensive muscle-building program that is highly effective and time efficient.

These exercises are performed on standard weight-stack machines that are available at almost all YMCAs, health clubs, and other fitness centers, and can

RECOMMENDED ROTARY AND LINEAR EXERCISES FOR THE MAJOR MUSCLE GROUPS

MUSCLE GROUP	BODY PART	ROTARY EXERCISE	LINEAR EXERCISE
Quadriceps	Front thighs	Leg Extension	Leg Press
Hamstrings	Rear thighs	Leg Curl	Leg Press
Pectoralis major	Chest	Chest Cross	Chest Press
Latissimus dorsi	Upper back	Pullover	Pulldown
Deltoids	Shoulders	Lateral Raise	Shoulder Press
Biceps	Front arms	Biceps Curl	Assisted Chinup
Triceps	Rear arms	Triceps Extension	Assisted Bar Dip
Erector spinae	Lower back	Lower Back Extension	—
Rectus abdominis	Midsection	Abdominal Curl	—

also be performed using dumbbells or a Bowflex apparatus in your home gym. Finding the appropriate exercise equipment should be relatively easy. The trickier part is learning to perform the exercises properly, productively, and safely. In Chapter 5, we present instructions and photographs of each strength-training exercise so that you can achieve the best muscle-building benefits.

LOOKING BACK . . . HINDSIGHT IS 20/20

Key strength-training guidelines for safe and effective muscle-building experiences can be summarized as follows:

Training frequency: Train 2 or 3 nonconsecutive days per week.

Training time: Schedule relatively brief sessions, typically 15 to 30 minutes in length, depending on the number of exercises performed.

Training sets: Perform one good set of each muscle-building exercise.

Training repetitions and resistance: Use an exercise resistance that permits successful performance of 8 to 12 controlled repetitions.

Training progression: Increase the exercise resistance by approximately 5 percent whenever 12 repetitions are completed in proper form two workouts in succession.

Training speed: Try to perform each repetition in about 6 seconds, taking 2 seconds to lift and 4 seconds to lower. Exercises with longer movement ranges will take longer to complete.

Training range: Try to perform each repetition through a full range of joint motion, being careful to avoid moving into painful positions.

Training posture: Stand and sit tall during your exercise performance.

Exercise breathing: Exhale during each lifting action, and inhale throughout each lowering action.

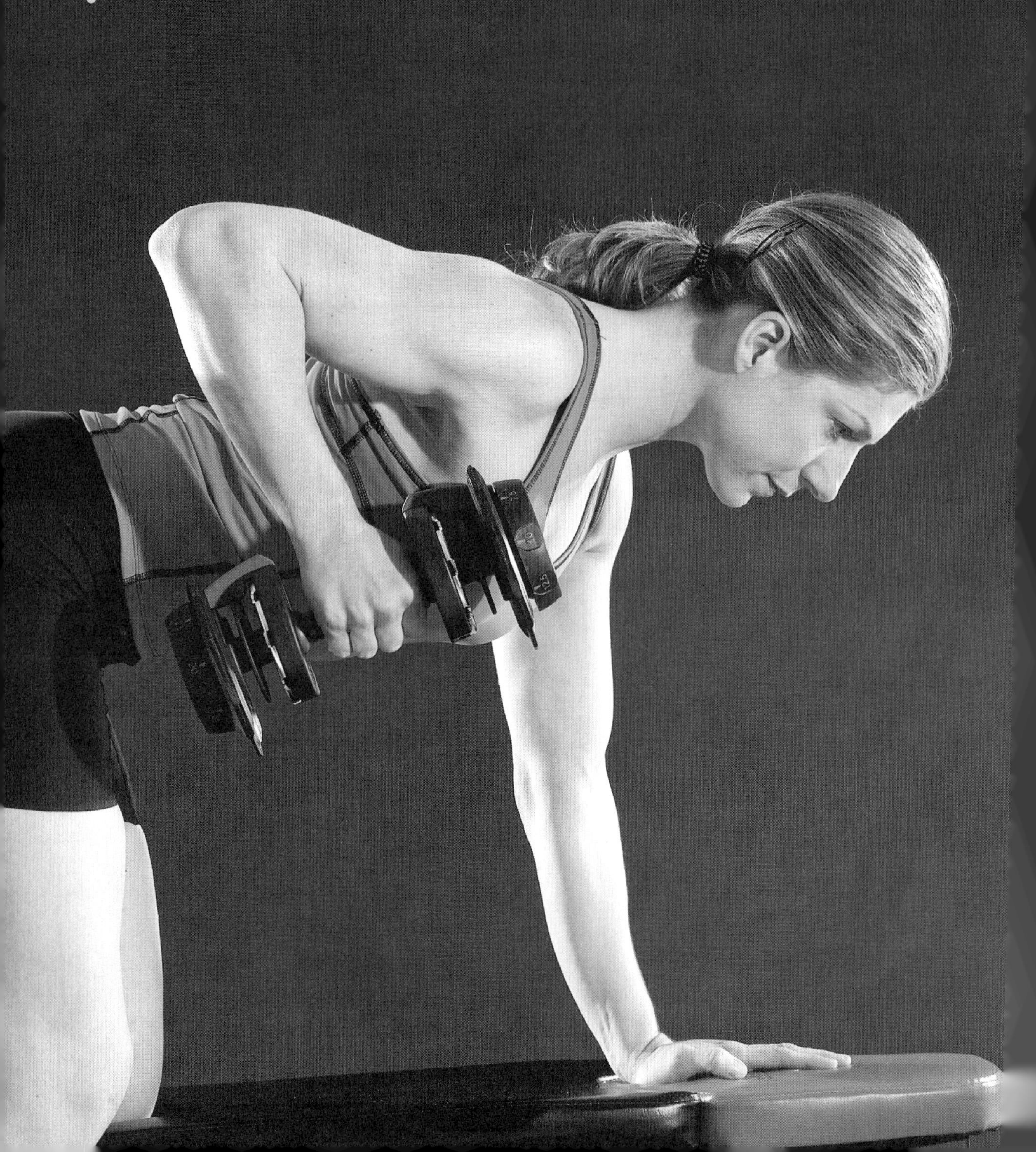

PART 2

THE GET STRONGER, FEEL YOUNGER PROGRAM

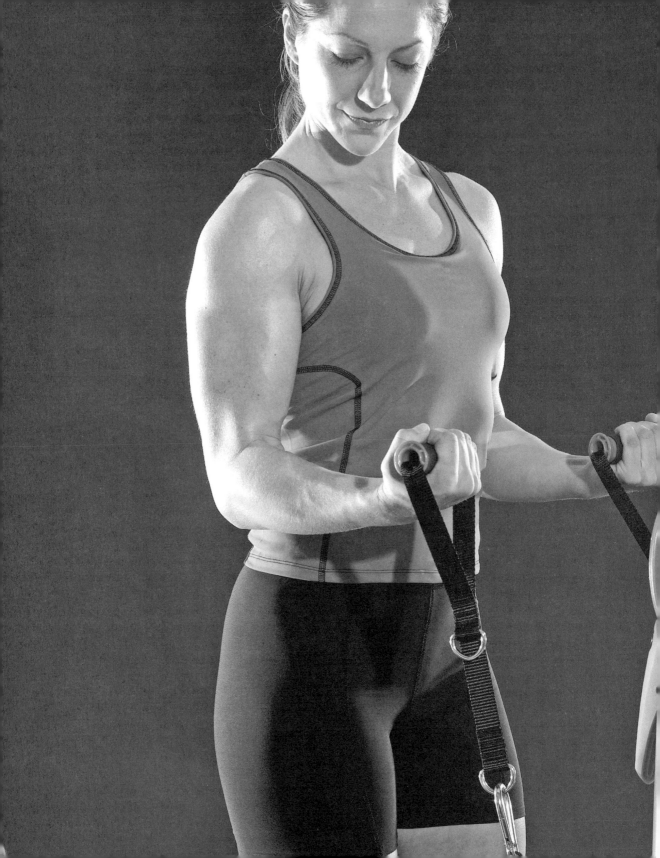

WHICH MUSCLES SHOULD I EXERCISE?

The main objective in selecting your strength-training exercises is to address all of your major muscle groups in the safest, most effective and efficient manner. With the exception of bodybuilders, weight lifters, and power athletes, most people in our time-pressured society prefer a basic and brief program of muscle-building exercises. In addition to fitting easily into a busy lifestyle, a shorter session using our recommended strength-training exercises may be more productive for muscle development than a more time-consuming and complex system of strength training. That's right: A shorter and more intense exercise session provides more muscle-building benefit than a longer and less intense training session.

We recently conducted a research study for one of the largest and best fitness chains in the United States. The corporate executives asked us to perform body composition assessments on more than 40 new members who chose to participate in one of two strength-training programs. One program option was a relatively short-duration workout (about 20 minutes) that involved a single set of each exercise. The other program option was a relatively long-duration workout of about 60 minutes that involved multiple sets of each exercise. Two out of three new members chose the shorter-duration strength-training program, whereas only one out of three chose the longer-duration workout option.

After 8 weeks, we reassessed all of the participants who completed their exercise program. Three out of four new members completed the shorter-duration strength-training program, whereas only two out of four new members completed the longer-duration exercise program.

Although the average fat loss was similar for both strength-training groups, the men and women who performed the shorter-duration exercise program developed twice as much muscle: 4.5 pounds compared with 2.0 pounds. How could this be? How could the participants who performed only 20 minutes of strength exercise lose as much fat and gain twice as much muscle as those who completed 60-minute strength-training workouts?

The answer to this question is directly related to training intensity. Unlike endurance-building activity that requires relatively low-effort exercise for relatively long periods of time (for example, walking, jogging, cycling), strength-building activity requires relatively high-effort exercise for relatively short periods of time (approximately 50 to 70 seconds). Brief bouts of high-effort exercise, referred to as high-intensity training, are best suited for muscle development. As the saying goes, you can train hard or you can train long, but you can't train hard for long. Most people can train hard for one set of each exercise but may progressively reduce their training intensity on repeat sets of the same exercise. For this reason, as well as for time efficiency, both our Standard Strength-Training Program and our Advanced Strength-Training Program require one properly executed set of each exercise. Of course, our Advanced

Strength-Training Program provides two successive exercises for each major muscle group, making it a more challenging and more productive exercise protocol.

For our purposes, a hard set of exercise is one that continues to the point of temporary muscle fatigue. Hard training sets are not characterized by poor form, jerky movements, or primal screams. You simply perform as many perfect repetitions as possible with a resistance that produces momentary muscle failure (fatigue) within 50 to 70 seconds (typically 8 to 12 repetitions). When you can't complete another lifting action, your set is over, and you move to the next exercise.

EXERCISE SELECTION

As we stated in Chapter 4, the key to muscular fitness is a basic and balanced strength-training program that addresses all of your major muscle groups. Of course, there are several exercise possibilities for each major muscle group and many equipment options with which to train. We recommend that you exercise at well-staffed and well-equipped fitness facilities. Most good fitness centers provide all of the recommended weight-stack machines needed for the exercises described and illustrated in the following section. We prefer training on biomechanically correct weight-stack machines because they provide for appropriate postural support, range control, and resistance control.

However, if you would rather train at home, this chapter also includes complete descriptions and clear photographs of our recommended exercises for home workouts. These exercises are performed with Bowflex equipment, dumbbells, elastic bands, and body-weight resistance.

For Fitness Facility Workouts Using Weight-Stack Machines

LEG EXTENSION

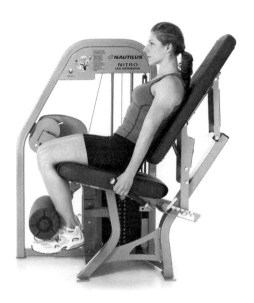
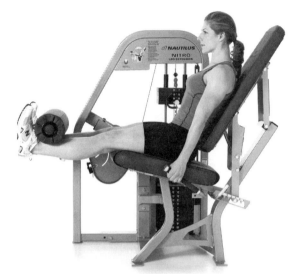

Starting Position: Sit on the machine with your knee joints directly in line with the machine's axis of rotation, your ankles under the movement pad, your knees flexed approximately 90 degrees, your hands on the handgrips, your back against the seat back, your head in a neutral (straight) position.

Ending Position: It's similar to the starting position except that your knees are extended approximately 180 degrees.

Action: Lift the movement pad until your legs are fully extended, completing the action in about 2 seconds. Pause momentarily in this position, then lower the movement pad until the weight stack almost touches, taking about 4 seconds. Repeat for 8 to 12 repetitions. Exhale during each upward leg movement and inhale throughout each downward leg movement.

Comment: *The leg extension exercise essentially isolates your quadriceps muscles. Be sure to complete each upward leg movement to the fully contracted (straight-leg) position.*

SEATED LEG CURL

Movement ROTARY

Muscles HAMSTRINGS (REAR THIGHS)

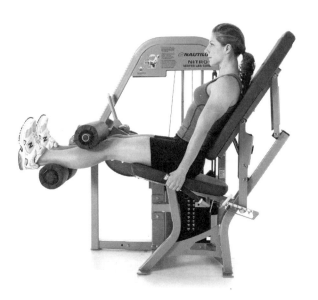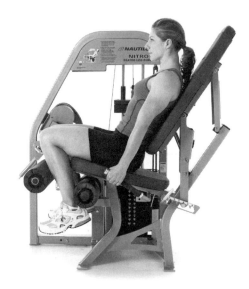

Starting Position: Sit on the machine with your knee joints directly in line with the machine's axis of rotation, your shins under the top movement pad, your ankles over the bottom movement pad, your knees extended approximately 180 degrees, your hands on the handgrips, your back against the seat back, your head in a neutral (straight) position.

Ending Position: It's similar to the starting position except that your knees are flexed approximately 60 degrees.

Action: Pull the movement pad downward until it touches the seat bottom, completing the action in about 2 seconds. Pause momentarily in this position, then raise the movement pad until the weight stack almost touches, taking about 4 seconds. Repeat for 8 to 12 repetitions. Exhale during each downward leg movement and inhale throughout each upward leg movement.

Comment: *The seated leg curl exercise essentially isolates your hamstring muscles. Be sure to perform each downward leg movement as far as the apparatus allows (knees flexed approximately 60 degrees).*

LEG PRESS

Movement   LINEAR

Muscles   QUADRICEPS (FRONT THIGHS), HAMSTRINGS (REAR THIGHS), GLUTEALS (BUTTOCKS)

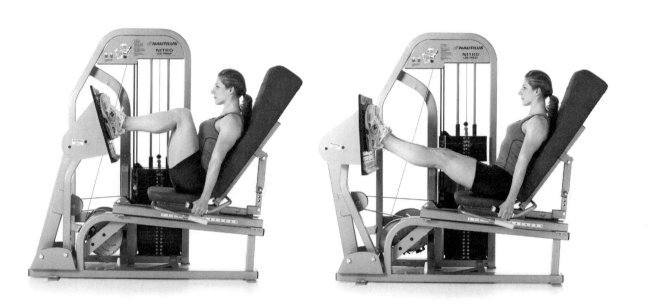

Starting Position: Sit on the machine with your feet evenly placed on the foot plate about hip-width apart, your shins parallel to the floor, your knees flexed approximately 90 degrees, your hands on the handgrips, your back against the seat back, your head in a neutral (straight) position.

Ending Position: It's similar to the starting position except that your knees are extended approximately 170 degrees.

Action: Press the foot plate forward until your legs are nearly extended, completing the action in about 2 seconds. Pause momentarily in this position, then return the foot plate backward until the weight stack almost touches, taking about 4 seconds. Repeat for 8 to 12 repetitions. Exhale during each forward leg movement and inhale throughout each backward leg movement.

Comment: *The leg press exercise involves concurrent contractions of the quadriceps, hamstring, and gluteal muscles. Be sure to stop each forward pressing action just short of the lockout position to avoid accidentally hyperextending your knee joint. If necessary, you may push your knees forward with your hands on the first repetition to initiate the movement of a relatively heavy weight stack.*

CHEST CROSS

Movement ROTARY

Muscles PECTORALIS MAJOR (CHEST)

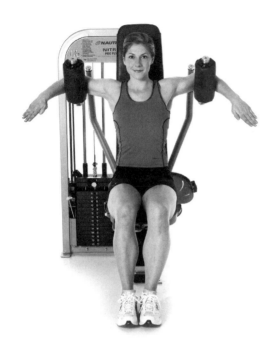 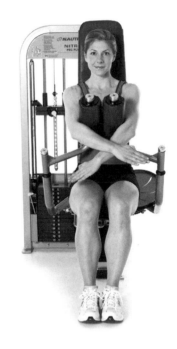

Starting Position: Sit on the machine with your back against the seat back, your arms behind widely separated movement pads, your shoulders in line with the machine's axes of rotation, your head in a neutral (straight) position.

Ending Position: It's similar to the starting position except that your arms are close together and the movement pads are contacting each other.

Action: Pull the movement pads downward until they make contact, completing the action in about 2 seconds. Pause momentarily in this position, then return the movement pads upward until the weight stack almost touches, taking about 4 seconds. Repeat for 8 to 12 repetitions. Exhale during each downward movement and inhale throughout each upward movement.

Comment: *The chest cross exercise basically isolates your pectoralis major muscles. Pull the movement pads all the way together on every repetition.*

CHEST PRESS

Movement LINEAR

Muscles PECTORALIS MAJOR (CHEST), ANTERIOR DELTOIDS (FRONT SHOULDERS), TRICEPS (REAR ARMS)

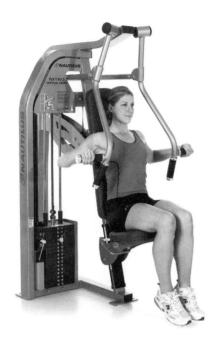 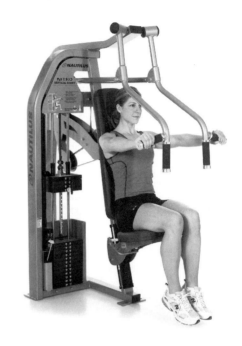

Starting Position: Sit on the machine with your back against the seat back, your hands on the handles, your elbows flexed approximately 75 degrees, your head in a neutral (straight) position.

Ending Position: It's similar to the starting position except that your elbows are extended forward approximately 180 degrees.

Action: Push the handles forward until your arms are extended, completing the action in about 2 seconds. Pause momentarily in this position, then return the handles backward until the weight stack almost touches, taking about 4 seconds. Repeat for 8 to 12 repetitions. Exhale during each forward arm movement and inhale throughout each backward arm movement.

Comment: *The chest press exercise involves concurrent contraction of the pectoralis major, anterior deltoid, and triceps muscles. Using the wider handles places more emphasis on your pectoralis major muscles and more stress on your shoulder joints. Using the narrower handles places more emphasis on triceps muscles and less stress on your shoulder joints. We recommend using the wider handles unless you experience shoulder discomfort.*

PULLOVER

Movement ROTARY

Muscles LATISSIMUS DORSI (UPPER BACK)

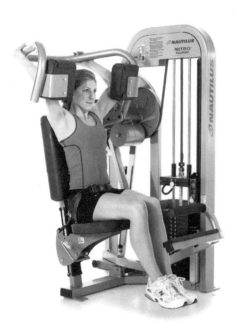
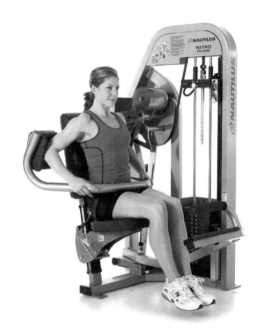

Starting Position: Sit on the machine with your back against the seat back, your elbows on the movement pads, your hands on the movement frame, your arms stretched comfortably overhead, your shoulders in line with the machine's axis of rotation, your head in a neutral (straight) position, and the seat belt buckled.

Ending Position: It's similar to the starting position except that your arms are along the sides and the movement frame is touching the seat belt.

Action: Pull the movement pads downward until the frame contacts the seat belt, completing the action in about 3 seconds. Pause momentarily in this position, then return the movement pads upward until the weight stack almost touches, taking about 5 seconds. Repeat for 8 to 12 repetitions. Exhale during each downward arm movement and inhale throughout each upward arm movement.

Comment: *The pullover exercise essentially isolates your latissimus dorsi muscles. Use the foot lever to adjust the movement pads for easy elbow entry and exit. Begin each repetition from a comfortably stretched arm position. The longer movement range of this exercise requires correspondingly longer movement times.*

PULLDOWN

Movement LINEAR

Muscles LATISSIMUS DORSI (UPPER BACK), BICEPS (FRONT ARMS)

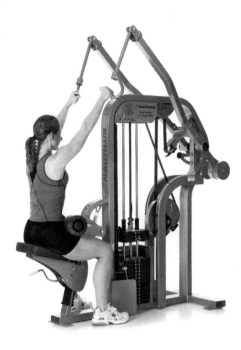
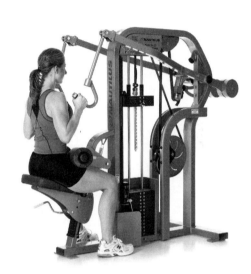

Starting Position: Sit on the machine with your torso erect, your thighs under the support pads, your hands on the handgrips, your arms fully extended upward, your head in a neutral (straight) position.

Ending Position: It's similar to the starting position except that your arms are flexed and the handles are below chin level.

Action: Pull the handles downward below chin level, completing the action in about 2 seconds. Pause momentarily in this position, then return the handles upward until the weight stack almost touches, taking about 4 seconds. Repeat for 8 to 12 repetitions. Exhale during each downward arm movement and inhale throughout each upward arm movement.

Comment: *The pulldown exercise involves concurrent contraction of the latissimus dorsi and biceps muscles. Keep your torso relatively erect throughout each repetition. Set the seat low enough so that your arms can stretch upward without the weight stack touching.*

LATERAL RAISE

Movement ROTARY

Muscles DELTOIDS (SHOULDERS)

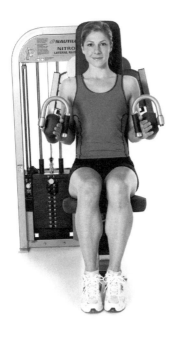
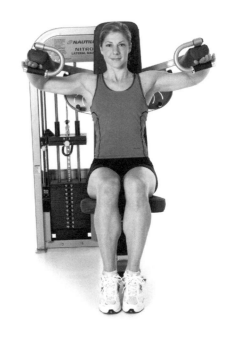

Starting Position: Sit on the machine with your back against the seat back, your shoulders in line with the machine's axes of rotation, your elbows against the movement pads, your arms against your sides, your head in a neutral (straight) position.

Ending Position: It's similar to the starting position except that your arms are horizontal, away from your sides.

Action: Lift the movement pads until your arms are parallel to the floor, completing the action in about 2 seconds. Pause momentarily in this position, then lower the movement pads until the weight stack almost touches, taking about 4 seconds. Repeat for 8 to 12 repetitions. Exhale during each upward arm movement and inhale throughout each downward arm movement.

Comment: *The lateral raise exercise essentially isolates your deltoid muscles. For best results, be sure to stop the upward movement when your arms are parallel to the floor.*

SHOULDER PRESS

Movement   LINEAR

Muscles   DELTOIDS (SHOULDERS), TRICEPS (REAR ARMS),
UPPER TRAPEZIUS (REAR NECK)

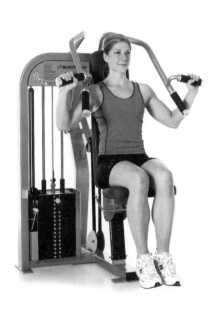 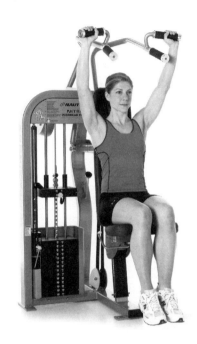

Starting Position: Sit on the machine with your back against the seat back, your hands on the handles, your elbows flexed approximately 75 degrees, your head in a neutral (straight) position.

Ending Position: It's similar to the starting position except that your elbows are extended upward approximately 180 degrees.

Action: Push the handles upward until your arms are extended, completing the action in about 2 seconds. Pause momentarily in this position, then return the handles downward until the weight stack almost touches, taking about 4 seconds. Repeat for 8 to 12 repetitions. Exhale during each upward arm movement and inhale throughout each downward arm movement.

Comment: *The shoulder press exercise involves concurrent contraction of the deltoid, triceps, and upper trapezius muscles. Using the wider handles places more emphasis on your deltoid muscles and more stress on your shoulder joints. Using the narrower handles places more emphasis on your triceps muscles and less stress on your shoulder joints. We recommend using the wider handles unless you experience shoulder discomfort.*

BICEPS CURL

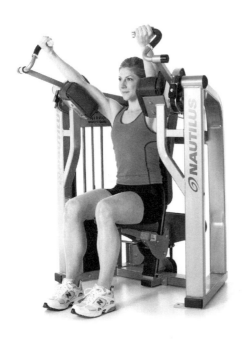 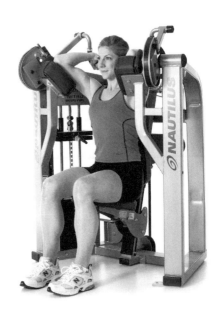

Starting Position: Sit on the machine with your back against the seat back, your elbows on the pads directly in line with the machine's axes of rotation, your arms slightly flexed (about 150 degrees), your hands on the handgrips (underhand grip), and your head in a neutral (straight) position.

Ending Position: It's similar to the starting position except that your elbows are fully flexed, approximately 30 degrees.

Action: Curl the handles backward as far as possible, completing the action in about 2 seconds. Pause momentarily in this position, then return the handles forward until the weight stack almost touches, taking about 4 seconds. Repeat for 8 to 12 repetitions. Exhale during each backward arm movement and inhale throughout each forward arm movement.

Comment: *The arm curl exercise essentially isolates your biceps muscles. To reduce the risk of elbow soreness, do not fully extend your arms during the forward movement. We recommend that you stop the downward movement at approximately 150 degrees of elbow extension when performing arm curls.*

WEIGHT-ASSISTED CHINUP

Movement LINEAR

Muscles LATISSIMUS DORSI (UPPER BACK), BICEPS (FRONT ARMS)

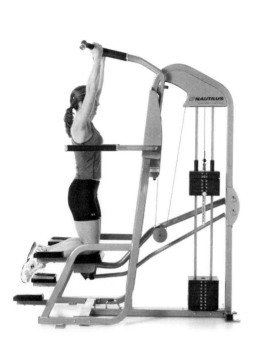 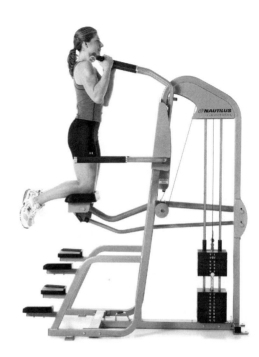

Starting Position: Kneel on the movement platform and hold the chin bar with an underhand grip, with your arms fully extended upward, your torso erect, and your head in a neutral (straight) position.

Ending Position: It's similar to the starting position except that your arms are flexed and your chin is above the bar.

Action: Pull your body upward until your chin is above the bar, completing the action in about 2 seconds. Pause momentarily in this position, then lower your body until your arms are fully extended, taking about 4 seconds. Repeat for 8 to 12 repetitions. Exhale during each upward body movement and inhale throughout each downward body movement.

Comment: *The assisted chinup exercise involves concurrent contraction of the latissimus dorsi and biceps muscles. Keep your torso straight throughout each repetition. Be sure to mount and dismount the movement platform in its top position. In this exercise, using more weight plates decreases the actual resistance, and using fewer weight plates increases the actual resistance.*

TRICEPS EXTENSION

Movement ROTARY

Muscles TRICEPS (REAR ARMS)

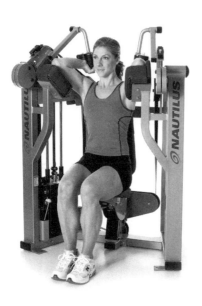
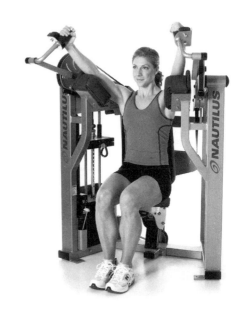

Starting Position: Sit on the machine with your back against the seat back, your elbows on the pads directly in line with the machine's axes of rotation and flexed approximately 60 degrees, your hands on the handgrips, and your head in a neutral (straight) position.

Ending Position: It's similar to the starting position except that your elbows are fully extended, approximately 180 degrees.

Action: Press the handles forward until your arms are essentially straight, completing the action in about 2 seconds. Pause momentarily in this position, then return the handles backward until the weight stack almost touches, taking about 4 seconds. Repeat for 8 to 12 repetitions. Exhale during each forward arm movement and inhale throughout each backward arm movement.

Comment: *The arm extension exercise essentially isolates your triceps muscles. To reduce the risk of elbow soreness, do not fully flex your arms during the backward movement. We recommend that you stop the backward movement at approximately 60 degrees of elbow flexion when performing arm extensions.*

WEIGHT-ASSISTED BAR DIP

Movement LINEAR

Muscles PECTORALIS MAJOR (CHEST), ANTERIOR DELTOIDS
(FRONT SHOULDERS), TRICEPS (REAR ARMS)

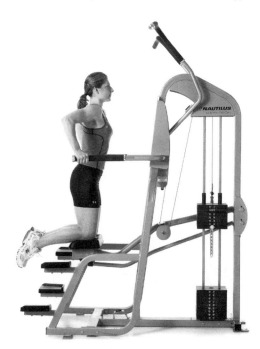 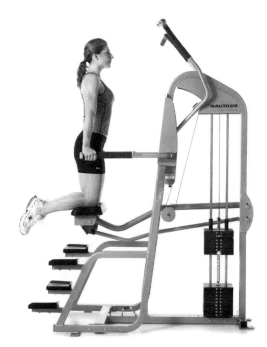

Starting Position: Kneel on the movement platform and grab the dip bars, with your elbows flexed approximately 90 degrees, your torso erect, and your head in a neutral (straight) position.

Ending Position: It's similar to the starting position except that your elbows are fully extended.

Action: Push your body upward until your arms are straight, completing the action in about 2 seconds.

Pause momentarily in this position, then lower your body until your elbows are flexed about 90 degrees, taking about 4 seconds. Repeat for 8 to 12 repetitions. Exhale during each upward body movement and inhale throughout each downward body movement.

Comment: *The assisted bar dip exercise involves concurrent contraction of the pectoralis major, anterior deltoid, and triceps muscles.*

Keep your torso straight throughout each repetition. Be sure to mount and dismount the movement platform in its up position. In this exercise, using more weight plates decreases the actual resistance, and using fewer weight plates increases the actual resistance. We recommend that you stop each lowering movement when your elbows reach 90 degrees of flexion.

LOWER BACK EXTENSION

Movement ROTARY

Muscles ERECTOR SPINAE (LOWER BACK)

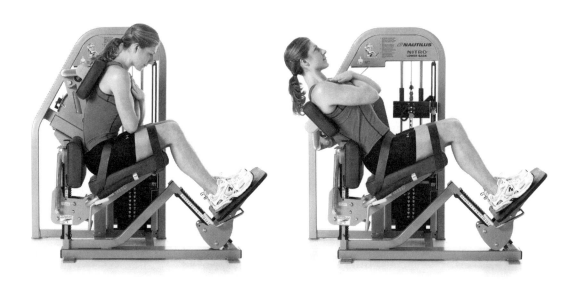

Starting Position: Sit on the machine with your hips against the seat back, the movement pad against the thickest part of your upper back, your arms crossing your chest, your feet on the foot plate, both seat belts buckled tightly, your trunk flexed forward approximately 50 degrees, and your head in a neutral (straight) position.

Ending Position: It's similar to the starting position

except that your trunk is extended backward approximately 120 degrees.

Action: Push the movement pad backward until it stops, completing the action in about 2 seconds. Pause momentarily in this position, then return the movement pad forward until the weight stack almost touches, taking about 4 seconds. Repeat for 8 to 12 repetitions. Exhale during each backward trunk movement and inhale

throughout each forward trunk movement.

Comment: *The lower back extension exercise, when performed properly, largely isolates your erector spinae muscles. Proper performance requires movement only in the trunk and not at the hip joint. This is best achieved by tightly securing both seat belts to keep your hips stabilized against the seat back. Keep your head in line with your torso throughout each repetition.*

ABDOMINAL CURL

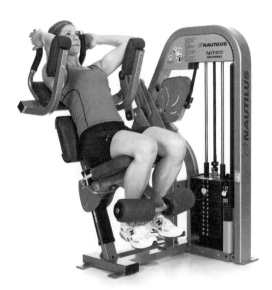 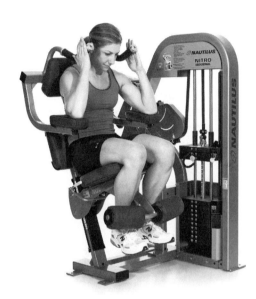

Starting Position: Sit on the machine with your hips against the seat back, the movement pad against the thickest part of the upper back, your elbows on the arm pads, your hands on the handgrips, your trunk extended backward approximately 120 degrees, and your head in a neutral (straight) position.

Ending Position: It's similar to the starting position except that your trunk is flexed forward approximately 50 degrees.

Action: Pull the movement pad forward until your abdominal muscles are fully contracted, completing the action in about 2 seconds. Pause momentarily in this position, then return the movement pad backward until the weight stack almost touches, taking about 4 seconds. Repeat for 8 to 12 repetitions. Exhale during each forward trunk movement and inhale throughout each backward trunk movement.

Comment: *The abdominal curl exercise, when performed properly, largely isolates your rectus abdominis muscles. Proper performance requires movement only in the trunk and not at the hip joint. This is best achieved by placing your feet behind the support pads and stopping the forward curling movement at about 50 degrees of trunk flexion. Keep your head in line with your torso throughout each repetition.*

ROTARY TORSO
(CLOCKWISE MOVEMENT)

Movement ROTARY

Muscles RIGHT INTERNAL OBLIQUES, LEFT EXTERNAL OBLIQUES
(SIDES OF MIDSECTION)

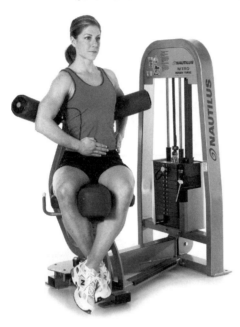 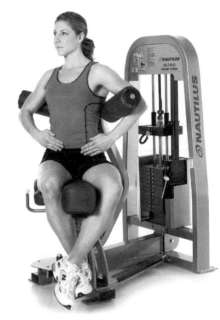

Starting Position: Sit on the machine with your hips against the seat ridge, your legs wrapped around the seat extension, your left arm behind the left arm pad, your right arm in front of the right arm pad, your torso erect, and your head in a neutral (straight) position. Set the machine at 30 degrees left of center.

Ending Position: It's similar to the starting position except that your torso is turned 30 degrees right of center.

Action: Move the arm pads through 60 degrees of clockwise movement, completing the action in about 2 seconds. Pause momentarily in this position, then return the arm pads counterclockwise until the weight stack almost touches, taking about 4 seconds. Repeat for 8 to 12 repetitions. Exhale during each clockwise movement and inhale throughout each counterclockwise movement.

Comment: *This exercise, when performed properly in the clockwise direction, involves concurrent contractions of your right internal and left external oblique muscles. Give equal effort pulling the left movement pad (with your left arm) and pushing the right movement pad (with your right arm), thereby placing equal stress on both sides of your torso. Keep your head in line with your torso throughout each repetition.*

ROTARY TORSO (COUNTERCLOCKWISE MOVEMENT)

Movement ROTARY

Muscles LEFT INTERNAL OBLIQUES, RIGHT EXTERNAL OBLIQUES (SIDES OF MIDSECTION)

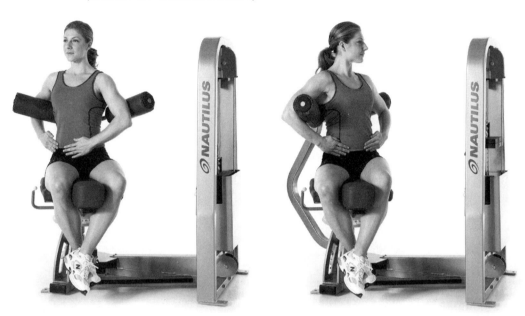

Starting Position: Sit on the machine with your hips against the seat ridge, your legs wrapped around the seat extension, your right arm behind the right arm pad, your left arm in front of the left arm pad, your torso erect, and your head in a neutral (straight) position. Set the machine at 30 degrees right of center.

Ending Position: It's similar to the starting position except that your torso is turned 30 degrees left of center.

Action: Move the arm pads through 60 degrees of counterclockwise movement, completing the action in about 2 seconds. Pause momentarily in this position, then return the arm pads clockwise until the weight stack almost touches, taking about 4 seconds. Repeat for 8 to 12 repetitions. Exhale during each counterclockwise movement and inhale throughout each clockwise movement.

Comment: *This exercise, when performed properly in the counterclockwise direction, involves concurrent contractions of your left internal and right external oblique muscles. Give equal effort pulling the right movement pad (with your right arm) and pushing the left movement pad (with your left arm), thereby placing equal stress on both sides of your torso. Keep your head in line with your torso throughout each repetition.*

For Home Workouts Using Dumbbells, Bands, and Body Weight

DUMBBELL STEPUP

Movement LINEAR

Muscles QUADRICEPS (FRONT THIGHS), HAMSTRINGS (REAR THIGHS), GLUTEALS (BUTTOCKS)

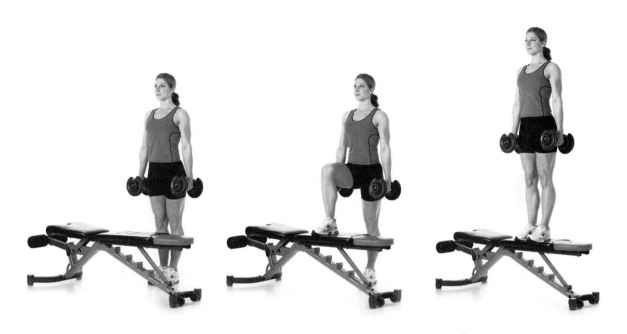

Starting Position: Stand in front of a stable bench, with both feet on the floor, your torso erect, your head in a neutral (straight) position, and your arms straight with dumbbells in your hands.

Ending Position: It's similar to the starting position except that both feet are on the bench.

Action: Step up first with your right foot, placing it securely on the bench, then step up with your left foot, placing it securely on the bench. Step down with your right foot, then step down with your left foot. Repeat for 8 to 12 repetitions. Exhale as you step up from the floor to the bench and inhale as you step down from the bench to the floor.

Comment: *The dumbbell stepup exercise involves concurrent contractions of the quadriceps, hamstring, and gluteal muscles. Be sure to maintain an erect posture throughout this exercise. Use a bench that is low enough for you to step on without lifting your knee higher than your hip (thigh parallel to the floor). When this exercise is repeated, step up first with your left foot followed by your right foot, and step down first with your left foot followed by your right foot.*

DUMBBELL SQUAT

Movement   LINEAR

Muscles   QUADRICEPS (FRONT THIGHS), HAMSTRINGS (REAR THIGHS), GLUTEALS (BUTTOCKS)

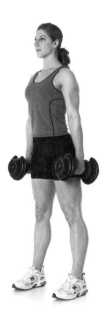 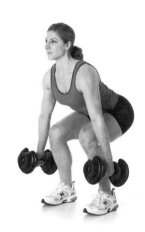

Starting Position: Stand with your feet about shoulder-width apart, your torso erect, your head in a neutral (straight) position, and your arms straight with dumbbells in your hands.

Ending Position: It's the same as the starting position with a momentary pause at the exercise midpoint when your thighs are parallel to the floor.

Action: Lower your hips downward and backward until your thighs are approximately parallel to the floor, completing the action in about 4 seconds. Return to the standing position, taking about 2 seconds. Repeat for 8 to 12 repetitions. Inhale during each downward movement and exhale throughout each upward movement.

Comment: *The dumbbell squat exercise involves concurrent contractions of the quadriceps, hamstring, and gluteal muscles. Be sure to maintain a relatively erect posture throughout this exercise, allowing for a slight forward bend at the hips in the down position. Do not let your knees move forward of your feet at any time during this exercise.*

DUMBBELL FLY

Movement ROTARY

Muscles PECTORALIS MAJOR (CHEST)

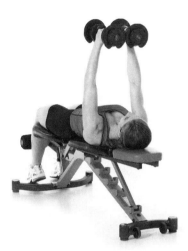
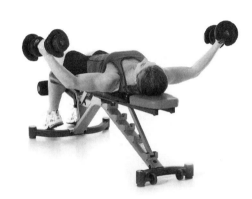

Starting Position: Lie faceup on a flat bench, with your feet on the floor, your arms extended directly above your chest, and dumbbells in your hands.

Ending Position: It's the same as the starting position, with a momentary pause at the exercise midpoint when your upper arms are parallel to the floor.

Action: Lower the dumbbells outward until your upper arms are approximately parallel to the floor, completing the action in about 4 seconds. Lift the dumbbells inward to the starting position, taking about 2 seconds. Repeat for 8 to 12 repetitions. Inhale during each downward movement and exhale throughout each upward movement.

Comment: *The dumbbell fly exercise basically isolates your pectoralis major muscles. To reduce the risk of injury, allow your elbows to bend (approximately 30 degrees) during the lowering phase of each repetition. Straighten your elbows during the lifting phase of each repetition.*

DUMBBELL BENCH PRESS

Movement LINEAR

Muscles PECTORALIS MAJOR (CHEST), ANTERIOR DELTOIDS (FRONT SHOULDERS), TRICEPS (REAR ARMS)

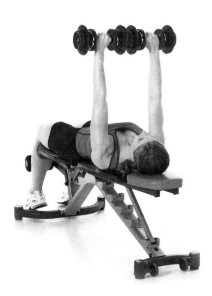
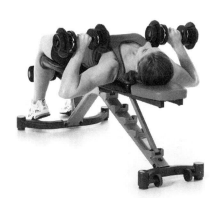

Starting Position: Lie faceup on a flat bench, with your feet on the floor, your arms extended directly above your chest, and dumbbells in your hands.

Ending Position: It's the same as the starting position, with a momentary pause at the exercise midpoint when the dumbbells contact the chest.

Action: Lower the dumbbells until they lightly contact your chest, completing the action in about 4 seconds. Press the dumbbells upward to the starting position, taking about 2 seconds. Repeat for 8 to 12 repetitions. Inhale during each downward movement and exhale throughout each upward movement.

Comment: *The dumbbell bench press exercise involves concurrent contractions of the pectoralis major, anterior deltoid, and triceps muscles. To emphasize the pectoralis major muscles, keep your elbows away from your sides as you perform the dumbbell bench press exercise.*

DUMBBELL PULLOVER

Movement ROTARY

Muscles LATISSIMUS DORSI (UPPER BACK)

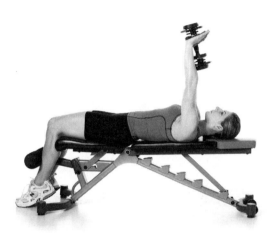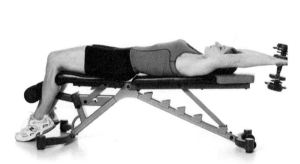

Starting Position: Lie faceup on a flat bench, with your feet on the floor, your arms extended directly above your chest, and both hands holding a single dumbbell.

Ending Position: It's the same as the starting position, with a momentary pause at the exercise midpoint when the dumbbell is at the lowest position behind your head.

Action: Lower the dumbbell backward behind the head as far as comfortable, completing the action in about 4 seconds. Lift the dumbbell upward and forward to the starting position, taking about 2 seconds. Repeat for 8 to 12 repetitions. Inhale during each downward movement and exhale throughout each upward movement.

Comment: *The dumbbell pullover exercise essentially isolates your latissimus dorsi muscles. Keep your elbows relatively straight throughout each repetition.*

DUMBBELL ROW

Movement LINEAR

Muscles LATISSIMUS DORSI (UPPER BACK), BICEPS (FRONT ARMS)

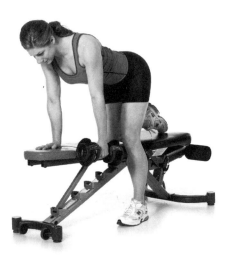 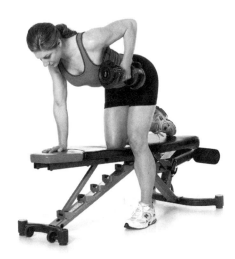

Starting Position: Stand with your left foot on the floor, your right knee and right hand on a bench, your back parallel to the floor, your head in a neutral (straight) position, and your left arm straight, holding a dumbbell.

Ending Position: It's the same as the starting position, with a momentary pause at the exercise midpoint when the dumbbell contacts the chest.

Action: Pull the dumbbell upward until it lightly contacts your chest, completing the action in about 2 seconds. Lower the dumbbell to the starting position, taking about 4 seconds. Repeat for 8 to 12 repetitions. Exhale during each upward movement and inhale throughout each downward movement.

Comment: *The dumbbell row exercise involves concurrent contractions of the latissimus dorsi and biceps muscles. To emphasize the latissimus dorsi muscles, keep your elbow close to your side as you perform the dumbbell row exercise. After completing a set of dumbbell rows with your left arm, place your left knee and left hand on the bench, and perform a set of dumbbell rows with your right arm. The purpose of placing one hand and one knee on the bench is to provide back support throughout this exercise.*

DUMBBELL LATERAL RAISE

Movement ROTARY

Muscles DELTOIDS (SHOULDERS)

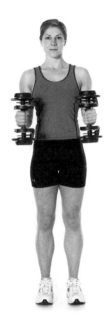 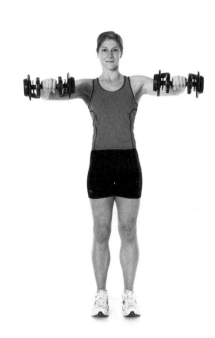

Starting Position: Stand with your feet about shoulder-width apart, your torso erect, your head in a neutral (straight) position, your elbows bent 90 degrees, your upper arms against your sides, your forearms parallel to the floor, with dumbbells in your hands.

Ending Position: It's the same as the starting position, with a momentary pause at the exercise midpoint when your upper arms are parallel to the floor.

Action: Lift the dumbbells upward and outward until your upper arms are parallel to the floor, completing the action in about 2 seconds. Pause momentarily, then lower the dumbbells to the starting position, taking about 4 seconds. Repeat for 8 to 12 repetitions. Exhale during each upward move-ment and inhale throughout each downward movement.

Comment: *The dumbbell lateral raise exercise essen-tially isolates your deltoid muscles. For best results, stop the upward movement when your upper arms are parallel to the floor. Be sure to keep your elbows at right angles throughout each repetition.*

DUMBBELL PRESS

Movement LINEAR

Muscles DELTOIDS (SHOULDERS), TRICEPS (REAR ARMS),
UPPER TRAPEZIUS (REAR NECK)

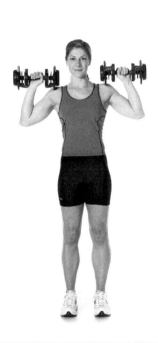
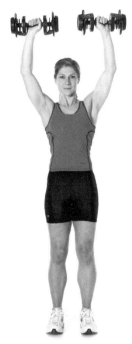

Starting Position: Stand with your feet about shoulder-width apart, your torso erect, your head in a neutral (straight) position, your elbows fully flexed, and with dumbbells in your hands directly above your shoulders.

Ending Position: It's the same as the starting position, with a momentary pause at the exercise midpoint when your arms are extended overhead.

Action: Press the dumbbells upward until your arms are extended overhead, completing the action in about 2 seconds. Lower the dumbbells to the starting position, taking about 4 seconds. Repeat for 8 to 12 repetitions. Exhale during each upward movement and inhale throughout each downward movement.

Comment: *The dumbbell press exercise involves concurrent contractions of the deltoid, triceps, and upper trapezius muscles. If you experience discomfort in your lower back or shoulder areas, perform dumbbell presses in an alternating manner (right arm, left arm, right arm, left arm).*

DUMBBELL BICEPS CURL

Movement ROTARY

Muscles BICEPS (FRONT ARMS)

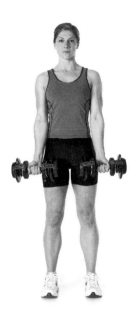 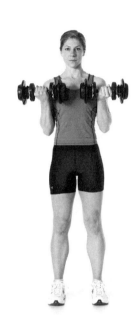

Starting Position: Stand with your feet about shoulder-width apart, your torso erect, your head in a neutral (straight) position, and your arms straight with dumbbells in your hands, palms facing forward.

Ending Position: It's the same as the starting position, with a momentary pause at the exercise midpoint when your elbows are fully flexed.

Action: Curl the dumbbells upward until your elbows are fully flexed, completing the action in about 2 seconds. Pause momentarily, then lower the dumbbells to the starting position, taking about 4 seconds. Repeat for 8 to 12 repetitions. Exhale during each upward move-ment and inhale throughout each downward movement.

Comment: *The dumbbell biceps curl exercise largely isolates your biceps muscles. For best results, keep your upper arms against your sides throughout each repetition.*

ELASTIC BAND DOOR PULL

Movement LINEAR

Muscles LATISSIMUS DORSI (UPPER BACK), BICEPS (FRONT ARMS)

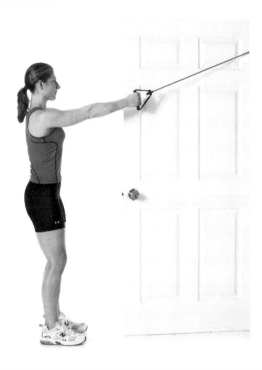
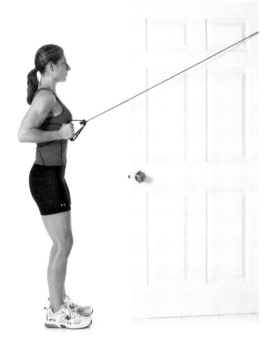

Starting Position: Place an elastic band over the top of a door, as shown. Stand with your feet about shoulder-width apart, your torso erect, your head in a neutral (straight) position, your arms extended upward and forward, and your hands holding the ends of the elastic band at a slightly stretched length.

Ending Position: It's the same as the starting position, with a momentary pause at the exercise midpoint when your hands are near your chest.

Action: Pull the ends of the elastic band downward and backward until your hands almost contact your chest, completing the action in about 2 seconds. Pause momentarily, then return the band to the starting position, taking about 4 seconds. Repeat for 8 to 12 repetitions. Exhale during each downward/backward movement and inhale throughout each upward/forward movement.

Comment: *The elastic band door pull exercise involves concurrent contraction of the latissimus dorsi and biceps muscles. For best results, keep your arms close to your sides as you perform the pulling action. You can increase the resistance by beginning with greater stretch on the elastic band, as well as by using progressively thicker bands.*

DUMBBELL TRICEPS EXTENSION

Movement ROTARY

Muscles TRICEPS (REAR ARMS)

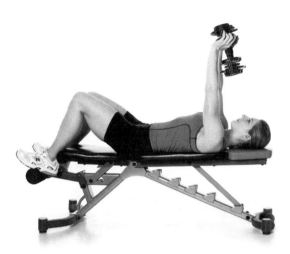
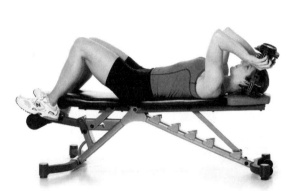

Starting Position: Lie faceup on a flat bench, with your feet on the floor or foot plate. Extend your arms directly above your head, and hold a dumbbell in each hand.

Ending Position: It's the same as the starting position, with a momentary pause at the exercise midpoint when the dumbbells are at their lowest position, beside the head.

Action: Lower the dumbbells backward beside your head, moving only your lower arms, completing the action in about 4 seconds. Raise the dumbbells to the starting position, moving only your lower arms, taking about 2 seconds. Repeat for 8 to 12 repetitions. Inhale during each downward movement and exhale throughout each upward movement.

Comment: *The dumbbell triceps extension exercise largely isolates your triceps muscles. For best results, keep your upper arms parallel to each other and vertical throughout each repetition.*

BODY-WEIGHT BENCH DIP

Movement LINEAR

Muscles PECTORALIS MAJOR (CHEST), ANTERIOR DELTOIDS (FRONT SHOULDERS), TRICEPS (REAR ARMS)

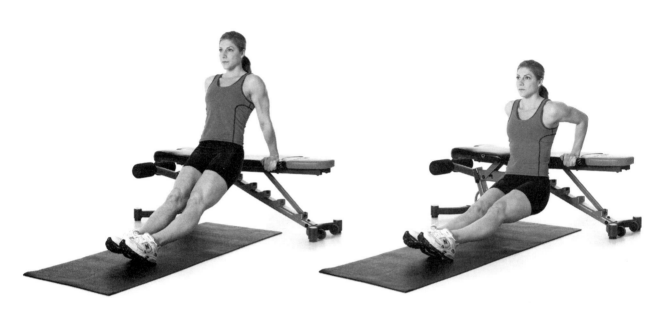

Starting Position: Assume a supported L position, with your heels on the floor, your arms extended and hands grasping the edge of a bench, your torso erect, and your head in a neutral (straight) position.

Ending Position: It's the same as the starting position, with a momentary pause at the exercise midpoint when your elbows are flexed to 90 degrees.

Action: Lower your hips in front of the bench until your elbows are flexed to approximately 90 degrees, completing the action in about 4 seconds. Press upward to the starting position, taking about 2 seconds. Repeat for 8 to 12 repetitions. Inhale during each downward movement and exhale throughout each upward movement.

Comment: *The body-weight bench dip exercise involves concurrent contractions of the pectoralis major, anterior deltoid, and triceps muscles. To emphasize the triceps muscles, keep the upper arms close to your sides throughout each repetition. To make this exercise more challenging, place your heels on a chair seat instead of on the floor. We recommend that you stop each lowering movement when your elbows reach 90 degrees of flexion.*

BODY-WEIGHT TRUNK EXTENSION

Movement ROTARY

Muscles ERECTOR SPINAE (LOWER BACK)

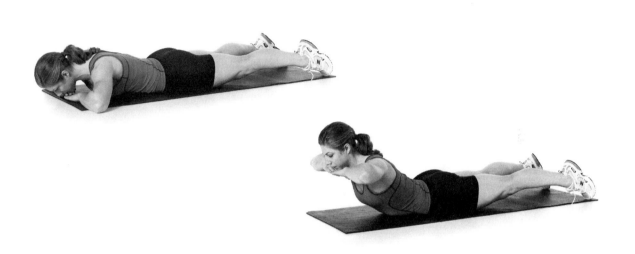

Starting Position: Lie facedown on a mat, with your hands folded under your chin and your head in a neutral (straight) position.

Ending Position: It's the same as the starting position, with a momentary pause at the exercise midpoint when your chest is farthest from the mat.

Action: Lift your chest off the mat as far as comfortable, completing the action in 1 to 2 seconds. Pause momentarily, then lower your chest to the mat, taking 2 to 4 seconds. Repeat for 8 to 12 repetitions. Exhale during each upward movement and inhale throughout each downward movement.

Comment: *The body-weight trunk extension exercise largely isolates the erector spinae muscles in your lower back. Although your chest will elevate only a few inches off the mat, you should feel a full contraction in the lower back extensor muscles. To make this exercise more challenging, you may extend your arms forward, rather than fold your hands under your chin.*

BODY-WEIGHT TRUNK CURL

Movement ROTARY

Muscles RECTUS ABDOMINIS (FRONT MIDSECTION)

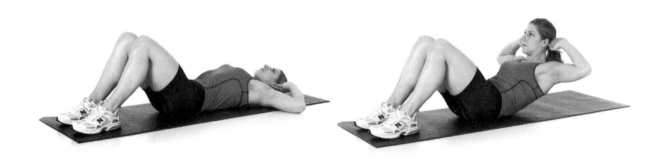

Starting Position: Lie faceup on a mat, with your hands folded behind your head, your head in a neutral (straight) position, your knees flexed approximately 90 degrees, and your feet on the floor.

Ending Position: It's the same as the starting position, with a momentary pause at the exercise midpoint when your upper back is farthest from the mat.

Action: Lift your upper back off the mat as far as comfortable, completing the action in 1 to 2 seconds. Pause momentarily, then lower your upper back to the mat, taking 2 to 4 seconds. Repeat for 8 to 12 repetitions. Exhale during each upward movement and inhale throughout each downward movement.

Comment: *The body-weight trunk curl exercise essentially isolates the rectus abdominis*

muscles in your front midsection. Although your upper back will elevate only a few inches off the mat, you should feel full contraction in the trunk flexor muscles. To make this exercise more challenging, you may perform additional repetitions or perform each repetition more slowly.

BODY-WEIGHT TRUNK CURL (ROTATION CLOCKWISE)

Movement ROTARY

Muscles LEFT EXTERNAL OBLIQUES (SIDE MIDSECTION), RIGHT INTERNAL OBLIQUES (SIDE MIDSECTION), RECTUS ABDOMINIS (FRONT MIDSECTION)

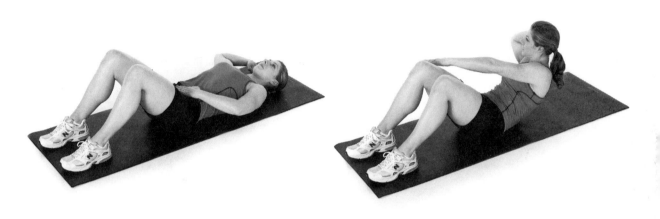

Starting Position: Lie faceup on a mat, with your right hand behind your head, your left hand on your stomach, and your head in a neutral (straight) position, your knees flexed approximately 90 degrees, and your feet on the floor.

Ending Position: It's the same as the starting position, with a momentary pause at the exercise midpoint when your left hand contacts your right knee.

Action: Lift your upper back off the mat as far as comfortable and turn your trunk clockwise so that your left hand contacts your right knee. These concurrent movements should take 1 to 2 seconds. Pause momentarily, then return to the starting position, taking 2 to 4 seconds. Exhale during each upward movement and inhale throughout each downward movement.

Comment: *This exercise involves concurrent contraction of the left external oblique, right internal oblique, and rectus abdominis muscles. Although your trunk will rotate clockwise only a few inches, you should feel full contraction in the activated oblique muscles. To make this exercise more challenging, you may perform additional repetitions or pause longer at the top (left hand to right knee) position.*

BODY-WEIGHT TRUNK CURL (ROTATION COUNTERCLOCKWISE)

Movement ROTARY

Muscles RIGHT EXTERNAL OBLIQUES (SIDE MIDSECTION),
LEFT INTERNAL OBLIQUES (SIDE MIDSECTION),
RECTUS ABDOMINIS (FRONT MIDSECTION)

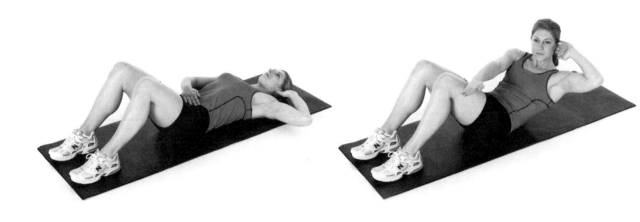

Starting Position: Lie faceup on a mat, with your left hand behind your head, your right hand on your stomach, and your head in a neutral (straight) position, your knees flexed approximately 90 degrees, and your feet on the floor.

Ending Position: It's the same as the starting position, with a momentary pause at the exercise midpoint when your right hand contacts your left knee.

Action: Lift your upper back off the mat as far as comfortable, and turn your trunk counterclockwise so that your right hand contacts your left knee. These concurrent movements should take 1 to 2 seconds. Pause momentarily, then return to the starting position, taking 2 to 4 seconds. Exhale during each upward movement and inhale throughout each downward movement.

Comment: *This exercise involves concurrent contraction of the right external oblique, left internal oblique, and rectus abdominis muscles. Although your trunk will rotate counterclockwise only a few inches, you should feel full contraction in the activated oblique muscles. To make this exercise more challenging, you may perform additional repetitions or pause longer at the top (right hand to left knee) position.*

For Home Workouts
Using Bowflex Apparatus

LEG EXTENSION

Movement **ROTARY**

Muscles **QUADRICEPS (FRONT THIGHS)**

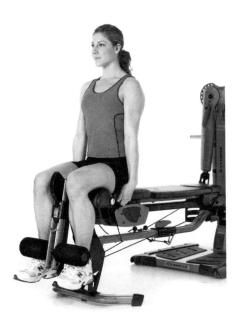 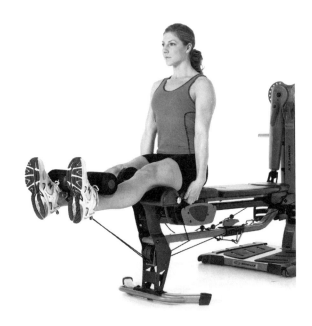

Starting Position: Sit on the bench with your knee joints directly in line with the axis of rotation, your ankles under the movement pad, your knees flexed approximately 90 degrees, your hands on the seat, your back straight, and your head in a neutral position.

Ending Position: It's similar to the starting position except that your knees are extended approximately 180 degrees.

Action: Lift the movement pad until your legs are fully extended, completing the action in about 2 seconds. Pause momentarily in this position, then lower the movement pad to the starting position, taking about 4 seconds. Repeat for 8 to 12 repetitions. Exhale during each upward leg movement and inhale throughout each downward leg movement.

Comment: *The leg extension exercise essentially isolates your quadriceps muscles. Make certain you complete each upward leg movement to the fully extended (straight leg) position.*

PRONE LEG CURL

Movement ROTARY

Muscles HAMSTRINGS (REAR THIGHS)

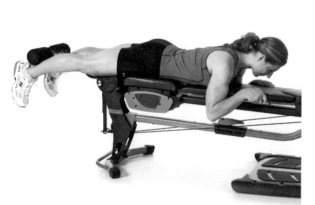
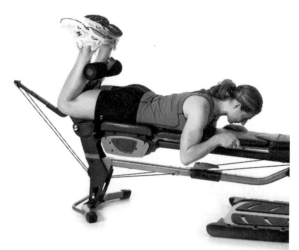

Starting Position: Lie facedown on the bench with your knee joints directly in line with the axis of rotation, your ankles under the movement pad, your knees extended approximately 180 degrees, your hands on the seat, and your head in a neutral position.

Ending Position: It's similar to the starting position except that your knees are flexed approximately 60 degrees.

Action: Pull the movement pad upward until it almost touches your buttocks, completing the action in about 2 seconds. Pause momentarily in this position, then lower the movement pad to the starting position, taking about 4 seconds. Repeat for 8 to 12 repetitions. Exhale during each upward leg movement and inhale throughout each downward leg movement.

Comment: *The prone leg curl exercise essentially isolates your hamstring muscles. Make certain you complete each upward leg movement to the fully contracted (pad almost touching buttocks) position.*

LEG PRESS

Movement LINEAR

Muscles QUADRICEPS (FRONT THIGHS), HAMSTRINGS (REAR THIGHS), GLUTEALS (BUTTOCKS)

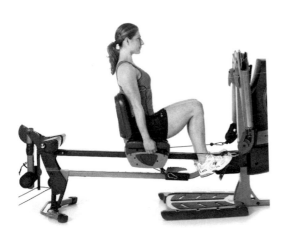 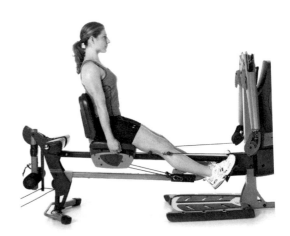

Starting Position: Sit on the sliding seat with your feet evenly placed on the foot plates, your knees flexed approximately 90 degrees, your hands on the seat, your back straight, and your head in a neutral position.

Ending Position: It's similar to the starting position except that your knees are extended approximately 170 degrees (just short of lockout position).

Action: Press the foot plates to move the sliding seat backward until your legs are nearly extended, completing the action in about 2 seconds. Pause momentarily in this position, then return to the starting position, taking about 4 seconds. Repeat for 8 to 12 repetitions. Exhale during each pushing movement and inhale throughout each return movement.

Comment: *The leg press exercise involves concurrent contractions of the quadriceps, hamstring, and gluteal muscles. Make certain you stop the pressing action just short of the lockout position to avoid accidentally hyperextending your knee joint.*

CHEST CROSS

Movement ROTARY

Muscles PECTORALIS MAJOR (CHEST)

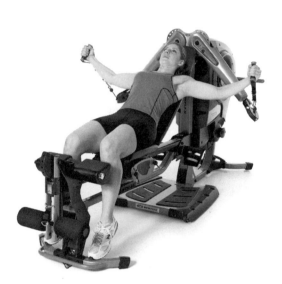 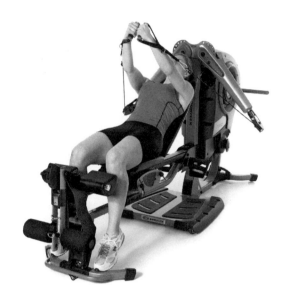

Starting Position: Sit on the machine with your back against the seat back, your arms extended sideward and parallel to the floor, your hands on the handgrips, your head in a neutral position, and your feet on the floor.

Ending Position: It's similar to the starting position except that your hands are touching.

Action: Pull the handgrips forward with a circular movement of your arms until your hands are together, completing the action in about 2 seconds. Pause momentarily in this position, then return to the starting position, taking about 4 seconds. Repeat for 8 to 12 repetitions. Exhale during each forward pulling movement and inhale throughout each return movement.

Comment: *The chest cross exercise basically isolates your pectoralis major muscles. Be sure to maintain relatively straight arms throughout the exercise set and to touch the handgrips on every repetition.*

CHEST PRESS

Movement LINEAR

Muscles PECTORALIS MAJOR (CHEST), ANTERIOR DELTOIDS
(FRONT SHOULDERS), TRICEPS (REAR ARMS)

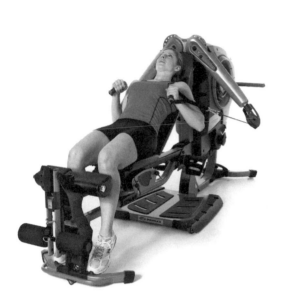 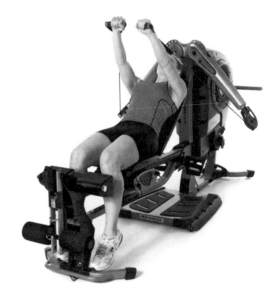

Starting Position: Sit on the machine with your back against the seat back, your hands on the handgrips by your chest, your elbows flexed approximately 30 degrees, and your head in a neutral position.

Ending Position: It's similar to the starting position except that your elbows are extended forward approximately 180 degrees.

Action: Push the handgrips forward until your arms are fully extended, completing the action in about 2 seconds. Pause momentarily in this position, then return to the starting position, taking about 4 seconds. Repeat for 8 to 12 repetitions. Exhale during each forward pushing movement and inhale throughout each return movement.

Comment: The chest press exercise involves concurrent contraction of the pectoralis major, anterior deltoid, and triceps muscles. Be sure to push the handgrips forward until your arms are fully extended and to return the handgrips no farther backward than your chest.

LATERAL FLY

Movement ROTARY

Muscles LATISSIMUS DORSI (UPPER BACK)

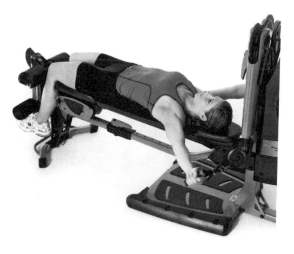 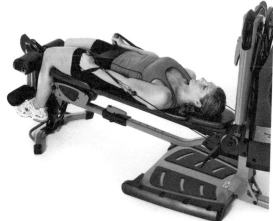

Starting Position: Lie faceup on a bench with your legs secured over the end of the bench, your hands on the handgrips, and your arms extended overhead in a V position.

Ending Position: It's similar to the starting position except that your arms are against your sides.

Action: Pull the handgrips forward to your thighs with your arms straight, completing the action in about 2 seconds. Pause momentarily in this position, then return to the starting position, taking about 4 seconds. Repeat for 8 to 12 repetitions. Exhale during each forward pulling movement and inhale throughout each return movement.

Comment: *The lateral fly exercise essentially isolates your latissimus dorsi muscles. Keep your elbows relatively straight throughout each repetition.*

SEATED ROW

Movement LINEAR

Muscles LATISSIMUS DORSI (UPPER BACK), BICEPS (FRONT ARMS)

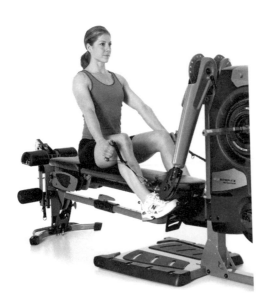
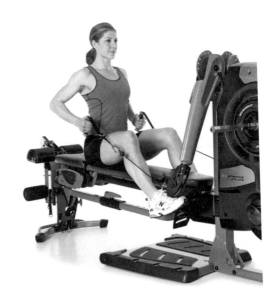

Starting Position: Sit on the machine with your torso erect, your arms extended forward, your hands on the handgrips, your head in a neutral position, and your feet on the foot plates.

Ending Position: It's similar to the starting position except that your elbows are flexed about 75 degrees with your hands by your sides.

Action: Pull the handgrips backward until your hands touch your sides, completing the action in about 2 seconds. Pause momentarily in this position, then return to the starting position, taking about 4 seconds. Repeat for 8 to 12 repetitions. Exhale during each backward pulling movement and inhale throughout each return movement.

Comment: *The seated row exercise concurrently works the latissimus dorsi and biceps muscles. Be sure to maintain an erect torso position throughout the exercise set.*

LATERAL RAISE

Movement ROTARY

Muscles DELTOIDS (SHOULDERS)

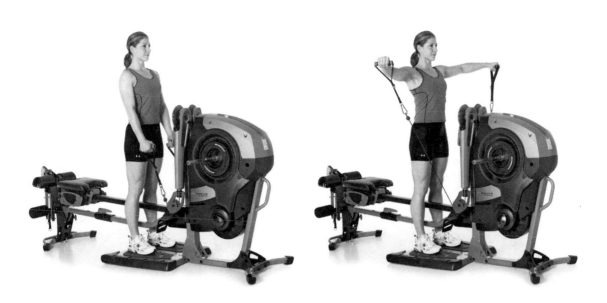

Starting Position: Stand tall, with your feet straddling the seat, your arms extended downward, your hands on the handgrips near your thighs, and your head in a neutral position.

Ending Position: It's similar to the starting position except that your arms are extended out to the sides, parallel to the floor.

Action: Lift the handgrips upward and sideward with a circular movement of your arms until your arms are parallel to the floor, completing the action in about 2 seconds. Pause momentarily in this position, then return to the starting position, taking about 4 seconds. Repeat for 8 to 12 repetitions. Exhale during each lifting movement and inhale throughout each lowering movement.

Comment: *The lateral raise exercise essentially isolates the deltoid muscles. Be sure to maintain an erect posture throughout the exercise set. Bend your elbows slightly during the lifting and lowering movements.*

SHOULDER PRESS

Movement LINEAR

Muscles DELTOIDS (SHOULDERS), TRICEPS (REAR ARMS),
UPPER TRAPEZIUS (REAR NECK)

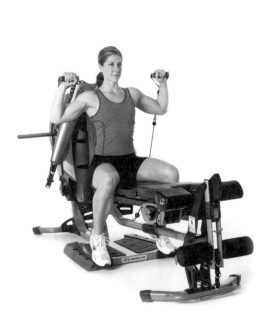 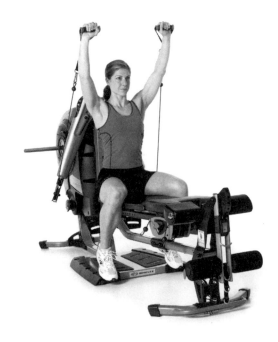

Starting Position: Sit on the machine with your back against the seat back, your elbows flexed approximately 60 degrees, your hands on the handgrips above your shoulders, your head in a neutral position, and your feet on the floor.

Ending Position: It's similar to the starting position except that your arms are extended above your shoulders.

Action: Push the handgrips upward until your arms are fully extended, completing the action in about 2 seconds. Pause momentarily in this position, then return to the starting position, taking about 4 seconds. Repeat for 8 to 12 repetitions. Exhale during each upward arm movement and inhale throughout each downward arm movement.

Comment: *The shoulder press exercise involves concurrent contraction of the deltoid, triceps, and upper trapezius muscles. Be sure to push the handgrips upward until your arms are fully extended and to return the handgrips just above your shoulders.*

BICEPS CURL

Movement ROTARY

Muscles BICEPS (FRONT ARMS)

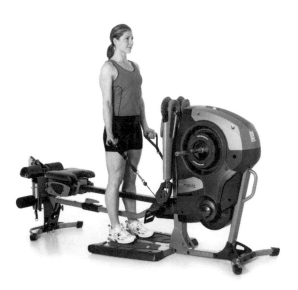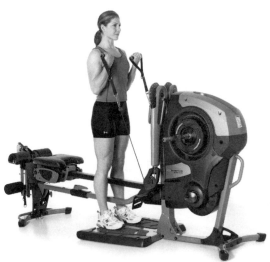

Starting Position: Stand tall, with your feet straddling the seat, your arms extended downward, your hands on the handgrips near your thighs, and your head in a neutral position.

Ending Position: It's similar to the starting position except that your elbows are flexed approximately 30 degrees with your hands by your chest.

Action: Curl the handgrips upward until your elbows are fully flexed, completing the action in about 2 seconds. Pause momentarily in this position, then return the handgrips to the starting position, taking about 4 seconds. Repeat for 8 to 12 repetitions. Exhale during each upward arm movement and inhale throughout each downward arm movement.

Comment: *The biceps curl exercise largely isolates your biceps muscles. Be sure to keep your upper arms against your sides throughout the performance of this exercise.*

PULLDOWN

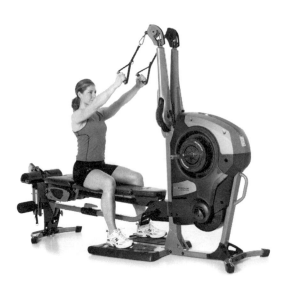 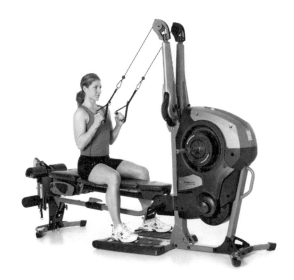

Starting Position: Sit on the machine with your torso erect, your arms extended upward, your hands on the handgrips with your palms facing each other, your head in a neutral position, and your feet on the floor.

Ending Position: It's similar to the starting position except that your elbows are flexed about 45 degrees with the handgrips below your chin.

Action: Pull the handgrips downward until they are below your chin, completing the action in about 2 seconds. Pause momentarily in this position, then return to the starting position, taking about 4 seconds. Repeat for 8 to 12 repetitions. Exhale during each downward pulling movement and inhale throughout each return movement.

Comment: *The pulldown exercise concurrently works the latissimus dorsi and biceps muscles. Be sure to maintain an erect torso position throughout the exercise set.*

TRICEPS EXTENSION

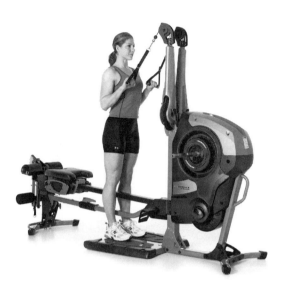
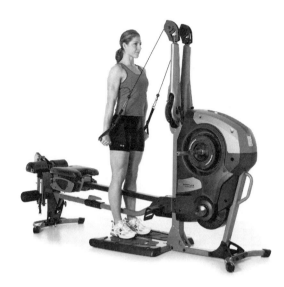

Starting Position: Stand tall, with your feet straddling the seat, your elbows flexed about 45 degrees, your hands at your chest and holding the handgrips with your palms facing away from you, and your head in a neutral position.

Ending Position: It's similar to the starting position except that your arms are fully extended downward.

Action: Extend your elbows until your arms are essentially straight down, completing the action in about 2 seconds. Pause momentarily in this position, then raise the handgrips to the starting position, taking about 4 seconds. Repeat for 8 to 12 repetitions. Exhale during each upward movement and inhale throughout each downward movement.

Comment: *The arm extension exercise essentially isolates your triceps muscles. Be sure to keep your upper arms against your sides throughout the performance of this exercise.*

LOWER BACK EXTENSION

Movement ROTARY

Muscles ERECTOR SPINAE (LOWER BACK)

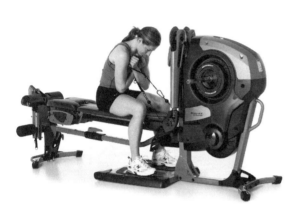 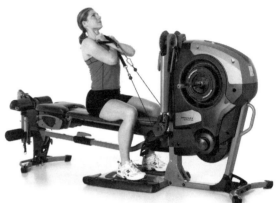

Starting Position: Sit on the machine, with your torso flexed forward approximately 50 degrees, your hands on the handgrips with arms crossed on the chest, your head in a neutral position, and your feet on the floor.

Ending Position: It's similar to the starting position except that your trunk is extended backward approximately 120 degrees.

Action: Extend your torso backward approximately 70 degrees while holding the handgrips on your chest, completing the action in about 2 seconds. Pause momentarily in the trunk-extended position, then return to the starting position, taking about 4 seconds. Repeat for 8 to 12 repetitions. Exhale during each backward trunk movement and inhale throughout each forward trunk movement.

Comment: *The lower back extension exercise, when performed properly, targets your erector spinae muscles. Do your best to keep your hips stationary and your arms crossed on your chest throughout the performance of this exercise.*

ABDOMINAL FLEXION

Movement ROTARY

Muscles RECTUS ABDOMINIS (FRONT MIDSECTION)

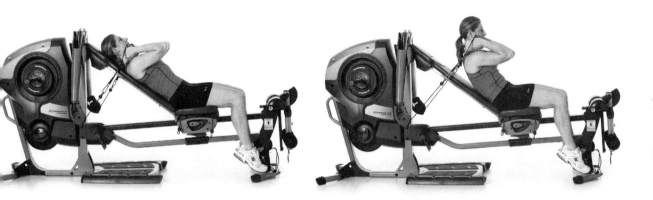

Starting Position: Sit on the machine with your back against the seat back, your hands on the handgrips on top of your shoulders, and your head in a neutral position.

Ending Position: It's similar to the starting position except that your trunk is flexed forward approximately 50 degrees.

Action: Curl your torso forward approximately 50 degrees while holding the handgrips on your chest, completing the action in about 2 seconds. Pause momentarily in the trunk-flexed position, then return to the starting position, taking about 4 seconds. Repeat for 8 to 12 repetitions. Exhale during each forward trunk movement and inhale throughout each backward trunk movement.

Comment: *The abdominal flexion exercise, when performed properly, targets your rectus abdominis muscles. Do your best to keep your hips stationary and your arms on top of your shoulders throughout the performance of this exercise.*

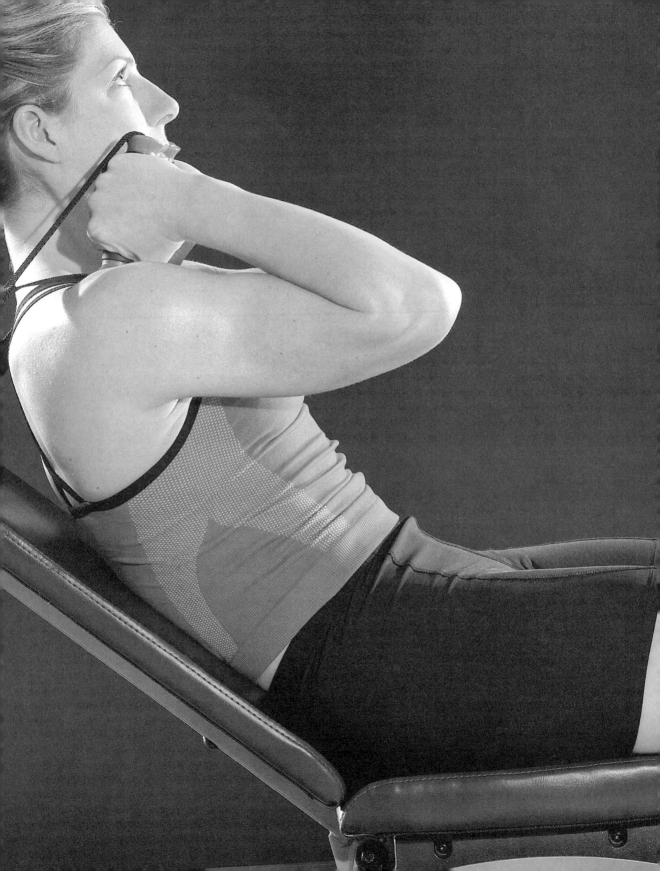

CHAPTER 6

HOW DO I START?

Getting off to a good start is the most important aspect of your muscle-building exercise program. A successful first step ensures the establishment of your new routine, plus you will be less likely to give up on the training process. The best advice we can give you is to start your strength training gradually and safely. At all costs, you must avoid making the following mistakes:

- Too much
- Too soon
- Too little
- Too heavy
- Too fast
- Too poor
- Too wrong

Unfortunately, most beginning exercisers turn their good intentions into poor judgments that can lead to overtraining, injuries, and discouragement. Let's take a look at the most common problems encountered by new strength trainers and how to prevent them.

TOO MUCH

Without question, the most prevalent and problematic characteristic of new trainees is trying to do too much. There is a misguided assumption that more strength training leads to better muscle-building results. While this approach may work for a small percentage of genetically gifted bodybuilders, long-duration and high-volume exercise sessions do more harm than good for beginners. Previously sedentary people simply do not respond well to long and arduous physical activity. Instead they tend to burn out, physiologically and psychologically, which usually results in discontinuation of their exercise program.

Our research study with new members at a large eastern United States fitness club chain demonstrated this outcome very clearly. One group of beginners performed three sets of 16 different exercises (high-volume training), while the other group of beginners completed just one set of 8 different exercises (low-volume training). After 8 weeks of training, only one-half of the high-volume exercise group was still training, whereas three-quarters of the low-volume exercise group was training regularly. Furthermore, those who completed the high-volume program added only 2 pounds of muscle, while those who completed the low-volume program gained more than 4 pounds of muscle.

Brief programs of strength exercise enable you to train hard, eliciting excellent strength gains and reducing your risk of overuse injuries. Long programs of strength exercise require lots of time, motivation, recovery ability, and injury resistance, which are uncommon characteristics in most people. It is important that you resolve that it is counterproductive to do too much strength exercise. Follow the program guidelines in this chapter, and try not to assume that more is better when it comes to strength training for fat loss.

TOO SOON

Although the familiar saying is "don't do too much too soon," we prefer to address these training problems separately. Gradual progression is the key to safe and successful muscle-building programs, especially with respect to positive physiological adaptations within your musculoskeletal system. Advancing your workouts too quickly is an invitation to injury that can be prevented by a sensible approach to strength/muscle building.

Muscle is a remarkable tissue that has the ability to shorten, lengthen, and produce widely varying levels of force. Muscle tissue also tends to be forgiving and resistant to injury. Unfortunately, other tissues that comprise our musculoskeletal system adapt more slowly to training stress and are more prone to damage. Progressing too quickly with strength training can be problematic for your tendons, ligaments, and connective tissue, especially when working the more vulnerable areas of your body, such as the shoulder joints.

Successful muscle building should be a lifetime activity that need not be hurried during the first few weeks of your program. Set realistic and progressive goals that can be attained in small steps over reasonable periods of time. For example, the first and most important goal of the Get Stronger, Feel Younger Plan is to schedule two or three weekly exercise sessions. Your second goal is to perform each workout to the best of your ability. If you do this and keep accurate training records, everything else should eventually fall into place. Don't try to rush your progress by doing too many exercises or using excessive weight loads. Your musculoskeletal system needs time to accommodate the increased physical demands of a sensible strength-building program.

TOO LITTLE

Before we continue to address the remaining series of *toos*, let us emphasize that it is also possible to do too little. Just as we should realize that advertisements that seem too good to be true usually are, we don't want to be misled by exceptionally easy exercise enticements. Claims that you can get fit in 5 minutes a day or that you can build muscle with extremely light resistance are generally untrue. Our studies with frail, elderly nursing home patients revealed outstanding results, but only when their physical therapists convinced them to use relatively heavy weight loads. Although they performed fewer exercises, these previously weak 90-year-old men and women followed essentially the same training guidelines as presented in the Get Stronger, Feel Younger Plan. Basic and brief exercise sessions work very well, as long as you use adequate training weight loads to stimulate the desired muscle development. You must realize that it will take a few weeks, not a few days, to see meaningful improvements.

TOO HEAVY

As we mentioned in the previous section, increasing your training weight load too much or too soon is a serious problem for many new exercisers. Generally speaking, too much resistance means any weight load increase that exceeds your previous training load by more than 5 percent. Your muscles rarely develop more than 5 percent greater strength between workouts, so it makes sense to keep your weight load increases below this level.

We recommend that you increase the number of repetitions before you increase the exercise resistance. First, select a weight load that enables you to complete 8 to 12 good repetitions. Let's say that you can presently perform nine leg presses with 50 pounds. Continue training with the 50-pound weight load until you can do 12 repetitions with proper form. At this point, you may increase the leg press weight load by 5 percent to 52.5 pounds. However, we advise that you be more patient and increase your training resistance only after you have performed 12 good repetitions on two consecutive workouts.

Following these guidelines should ensure safe and successful muscle-building experiences that provide a solid base for you to progressively increase your exercise weight loads. It is always better to feel that your training resistance was too light for one workout, rather than to regret that it was too heavy.

TOO FAST

In our opinion, the most potentially harmful problem among new exercisers is training too fast. Moving too quickly through a repetition reduces your muscle-building stimulus and raises your risk of injury. While you cannot produce as much muscle force or muscle tension with fast repetitions, you can place more injury-related stress on your joints. Consequently, fast movement speeds are counterproductive for muscle development and inhibit exercise safety.

As we mentioned in Chapter 4, we recommend slow to moderate repetition speeds, taking approximately 6 seconds to complete each repetition. We advise that you perform the lifting movement in about 2 seconds and the lowering movement in about 4 seconds. This training method provides an effective muscle-building stimulus during each phase (up and down) of your repetitions.

Training at faster speeds also emphasizes momentum as a catalyst for movement rather than muscle effort. Quick lifting actions are characterized by too much joint stress at the beginning of the repetition and too little muscle tension throughout the remainder of the repetition. Although this type of momentum-assisted strength training may enable you to use heavier weight loads, the disadvantages in the form of unnecessary impact force and excess joint stress far outweigh any perceived benefits. For best short-term and long-term results, train under control with relatively slow repetition speeds.

TOO POOR

The *too poor* category includes all types of improper training techniques such as breath holding, poor posture, and body contortions, as well as fast movement speeds and short movement ranges. Never hold your breath when performing strength exercise because this can cause a sharp rise in blood pressure. Breathe out (exhale) during each lifting action, and breathe in (inhale) during each lowering action. Sit or stand tall throughout each training set without

(continued on page 96)

PRETRAINING PROGRAM FOR PEOPLE WITH GENERAL OR SPECIFIC AREAS OF WEAKNESS

Due to age, injury, illness, or other factors, some individuals have too little overall muscle strength to effectively engage in our beginner training program. For example, there are people who are simply so weak that they cannot successfully perform a standard-length exercise program. There are others who have an acceptable level of overall muscle strength, but have a weak area (such as a bad back or recent knee surgery) and must therefore modify their exercise program accordingly. Finally, some people may be injury free, but have a disease or condition (such as osteoporosis or arthritis) that requires more individualized introductory exercise sessions. To prevent further problems and to facilitate productive muscle-building experiences, we recommend a pretraining preparation program to strengthen the vulnerable areas of the body first.

This abbreviated training program is designed to strengthen the weaker links in your body's musculoskeletal system, thereby reducing the risk of injury (such as lower back pain) and establishing a firm foundation for overall muscle development. We recom-mend at least 4 weeks of the pretraining program prior to participating in our standard beginning muscle-building program for those individuals with low overall or specific strength levels. Just be sure to check with your personal physician prior to performing this or any other exercise program.

Pretraining Exercise Guidelines

1. Perform one set of each exercise.

2. Use a resistance that permits 8 to 12 carefully controlled repetitions.

3. Perform each repetition in approximately 6 seconds, using 2 seconds for each lifting action and 4 seconds for each lowering action.

4. Exhale during lifting actions and inhale throughout lowering actions.

5. Use a full range of movement if possible, but do not move into uncomfortable positions.

6. Increase the weight load by no more than 5 percent (1-pound weight increments are fine) when 12 repetitions can be

completed with good form on two consecutive workouts.

7. Train 2 or 3 nonconsecutive days each week.

Sample Pretraining Exercise Program for Lower Back Weakness

The pretraining program features three exercises for the core musculature (all of your midsection muscles), namely the lower back machine for your erector spinae muscles, the abdominal machine for your rectus abdominis muscles, and the rotary torso machine for your oblique muscles. Although you may approach the pretraining program in other ways, the following represents a sample exercise session for people who experience lower back weakness.

Warmup

■ 5 or more minutes of easy pedaling on a recumbent or upright exercise cycle

Workout

■ One set of 8 to 12 repetitions on the lower back machine or the Body-Weight Trunk Extension exercise

■ One set of 8 to 12 repetitions on the abdominal machine or the Body-Weight Trunk Curl exercise

■ One set of 8 to 12 repetitions each direction on the rotary torso machine or the Body-Weight Trunk Curl Rotation exercise

Cooldown

■ 5 or more minutes of easy pedaling on a recumbent or upright exercise cycle

Although such a brief training session may not seem worth the effort of traveling to the fitness center (perhaps you've tried before and failed), be assured that this approach can work. A several-year study at the University of Florida College of Medicine showed an 80 percent success rate (significantly less discomfort) with lower back pain patients who performed just one set of lower back extensions, 2 or 3 days a week, for a period of 10 weeks. When performed properly and regularly, a little muscle-building exercise can go a long way. Keep in mind that you must first overcome limiting muscle weaknesses in order to successfully perform overall muscle-building exercises that will facilitate fat loss.

slouching forward, leaning backward, or tilting to one side. Be sure to use seat belts where provided to maintain proper body alignment during the exercise performance.

Try to avoid body contortions, commonly referred to as squirms, because these inappropriate actions can lead to serious injuries. Squirms are typically ill-fated attempts to gain a leverage advantage for completing an extra repetition. It is much better to perform 10 good repetitions than to squirm your way through an 11th repetition and injure yourself in the process.

We have repeatedly found that people who emphasize proper exercise form experience better training results and fewer training setbacks than those who pay less attention to their exercise technique. We encourage you to make every repetition as productive as possible by using proper training techniques and avoiding sloppy exercise execution.

TOO WRONG

Too many new exercisers set the wrong goals for their fitness program and, therefore, never attain them. Worse yet, they become discouraged and discontinue their training program altogether. Goals such as simply "getting in shape" or just "losing weight" are too vague to measure in any meaningful manner. Instead, you need to address the most important and specific objectives of your exercise program, which are to build/replace muscle and to increase your metabolism so that you can successfully reduce fat, maintain a healthy body composition, and enjoy a physically fit appearance.

Even people who set appropriate training objectives typically have the wrong plan for achieving them. They tend to listen to the wrong advice, such as performing hundreds of repetitions of highly ineffective exercises. These include some popular calisthenics such as endless situps, side bends, and assorted tummy wiggles, which usually lead the list, as well as hours of aerobic activities that do not elicit muscle growth or enhance your resting metabolism.

Then there is the problem of wrong measurement. Most diet plans live and die by the numbers displayed on the bathroom scale. Unfortunately, this is a very inaccurate and imprecise assessment of the true change in terms of body composition. Remember that you need to concurrently add muscle and reduce fat. This combination of beneficial outcomes may not show as much weight loss on the scale. Consider that you should gain about 3 pounds of muscle and lose at least 9 pounds of fat during your first 10 weeks on our plan if you follow the program correctly. This represents only a 6-pound decrease in scale weight, but is actually a 12-pound improvement in body composition, physical fitness, and personal appearance. As you can see, scales may give only half-truths, so be sure to have a fitness professional periodically check your body composition changes with skinfold calipers or similar assessment technologies. We recommend working with fitness instructors/personal trainers who have a nationally recognized professional certification, such as the following:

- American Council on Exercise (ACE)
- American College of Sports Medicine (ACSM)
- Cooper Institute
- International Fitness Professionals Association (IFPA)
- National Academy of Sports Medicine (NASM)
- National Strength and Conditioning Association (NSCA)
- National Strength Professionals Association (NSPA)
- Young Men's Christian Association (YMCA)

Finally, most new exercisers make the mistake of neglecting to keep careful records of their training program. They want to get in shape as quickly as possible, and they feel that any type of exercise will achieve that objective. Of course, they are wrong. They need to understand that a well-designed, systematic, and progressive program of muscle-building exercise is essential for permanent fat loss and that careful recording of each training session facilitates achievement of this goal.

REVIEW OF THE "TOO"

- **Too much:** Without question, the most prevalent and problematic characteristic of new trainees is trying to do too much.

- **Too soon:** Gradual progression is the key to safe and successful muscle-building programs, especially with respect to positive physiological adaptations within your musculoskeletal system.

- **Too little:** Claims that you can get fit in 5 minutes a day or build muscle with extremely light resistance are generally untrue.

- **Too heavy:** Generally speaking, too much resistance means any weight load increase that exceeds your previous training load by more than 5 percent.

- **Too fast:** Moving too quickly through a repetition reduces your muscle-building stimulus and raises your risk of injury.

- **Too poor:** This category includes all types of improper training techniques such as breath holding, poor posture, and body contortions, as well as fast movement speeds and short movement ranges.

- **Too wrong:** Too many new exercisers set the wrong goals for their fitness program and, therefore, never attain them.

One of your authors and his wife serve as good examples of some of the *too* problems. Wayne has always had a habit of doing *too much*, *too soon*, with *too heavy* weight loads. Consequently, he has frequently encountered unnecessary aches and pains, as well as occasional injuries, due to stressing his musculoskeletal system beyond its recovery abilities.

On the other hand, Wayne's wife, Claudia, tends to be *too conservative* with her personal program of strength exercise. Although she trains on a regular basis, Wayne considers her workouts *too brief* and her weight loads *too light* to fully develop her muscular potential. Of course, Claudia likes her concise and comfortable training program, feels it provides plenty of muscle strength for working with her horses, and notes that she has no exercise-related injuries. Perhaps if Wayne trained a little more like Claudia, and Claudia trained a little more like Wayne, they would both experience better results.

REALITY CHECK

We all need to assess where we stand on the genetics gifts scale, physiologically speaking. A very small percentage of people are gifted with exceptionally strong and extremely responsive musculoskeletal systems. These few individuals have the physical ability to train both hard and long without breaking down.

Unfortunately, most of us are not in this category. We cannot consistently perform high-volume and long-duration weight workouts without encountering physiological breakdown and experiencing a variety of overuse injuries. We need to train in a different manner to safely and successfully attain our genetic potential.

The Standard Strength-Training Program presented in Chapter 7 is perfect for most women who want to get stronger and feel younger. In fact, when performed properly and progressively, these exercise protocols will bring you pretty close to your genetic potential for muscular development and strength fitness. If you discover that you have the interest and ability to make additional strength gains, the Advanced Strength-Training Program in Chapter 8 should be highly effective for making further progress.

Both our Standard and Advanced Strength-Training Programs feature productive exercises and research-based workouts that maximize your muscular fitness and minimize your training time. Just be sure to apply the exercise guidelines presented in this chapter to achieve your best training results.

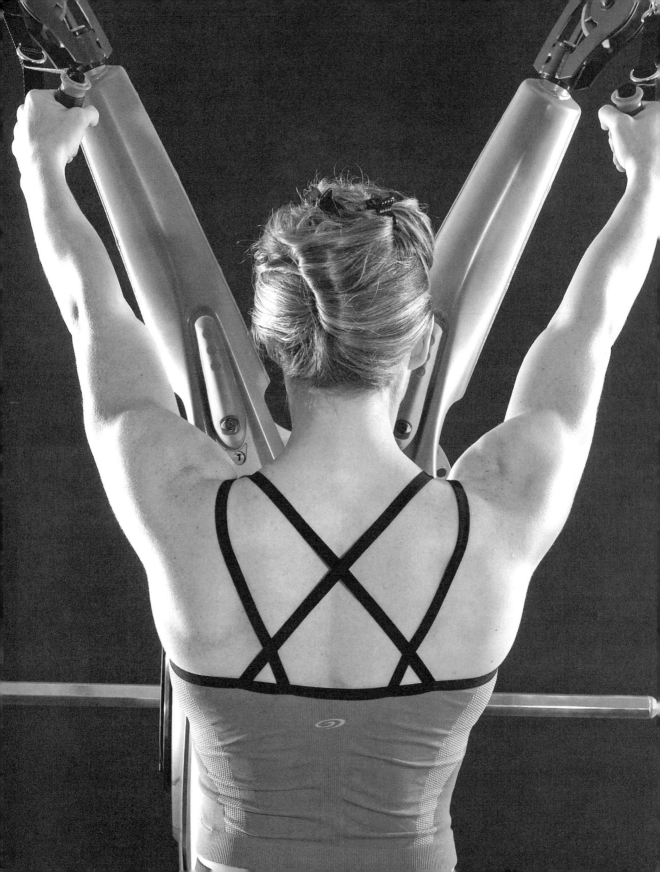

CHAPTER 7

MUSCLE-BUILDING PROGRAM FOR NEW EXERCISERS

The Standard Strength-Training Program is designed for people who want to restore their strength, build their muscle, increase their metabolism, and reduce their body fat. The Get Stronger, Feel Younger Plan is not a temporary "food diet" of caloric restrictions, but a permanent *activity diet* of muscle-building exercises that will improve your body composition and physical fitness for life.

Of course, you can implement the program at home with barbells, dumbbells, elastic bands, or a Bowflex apparatus. However, we know that most of you will be more successful training on your own after you've learned proper exercise performance and developed a personal exercise habit at a well-equipped and well-instructed fitness center. You should have little difficulty finding a fitness facility that provides the exercise equipment recommended here, as well as professional instructors to educate and motivate you. Working with qualified fitness instructors until you develop the competence and confidence to exercise on your own is a valuable first step on the road to improved fitness.

If your strength-training facility does not have all of the weight-stack machines featured here, your instructor can make appropriate substitutions of similar exercises. If your instructor suggests a slightly different exercise, that is acceptable as long as the adjustments are minor. However, try not to stray too far from the program or training protocol. Major changes in our well-researched recommended exercise plan may prove less effective, especially protocols that require more training exercises, more training sets, higher training volumes, heavier or lighter exercise weight loads, more or fewer exercise repetitions, faster training speeds, and more frequent training sessions. Our studies demonstrate that safe and successful muscle-building programs for new exercisers are characterized by basic and brief strength-training sessions, and recent research supports this type of training for advanced exercisers as well.

Your instructor may suggest a few minutes of aerobic activity (treadmill walking, stationary cycling, and so forth) as a warmup and a cooldown before and after your muscle-building workout. This is fine, but just be sure not to overdo the intensity or duration of your warmup and cooldown segments. Five to 10 minutes of each at a comfortable pace should be more than sufficient.

Some instructors may advise you to add equal amounts of endurance exercise to your muscle-building program. This is also fine; just be sure to start slowly and progress gradually, working up to approximately 20 to 30 minutes of endurance exercise at a moderate effort level. Keep in mind that the muscle-building activity has far more impact on your fat loss and physical appearance, so make this your primary physical activity.

A BASIC AND EFFICIENT PLAN

If you are a new exerciser in at least fair physical condition and have your physician's approval to perform muscle-building exercise, our Standard Strength-Training Program is the plan you should perform on a regular basis.

Although you do not need to follow this program precisely to attain body composition benefits, our 15 years of research studies indicate that you will achieve the best results by performing these exercises as presented and progressing according to the training guidelines. With few exceptions, you should neither add to nor subtract from the recommended exercise protocol. Quite simply, if you follow the program without doing more or doing less, you should experience excellent results and see consistent improvements in your body composition, physical fitness, and personal appearance. Your clothes will fit better, you'll have more energy, and you'll be able to perform everyday tasks with greater ease and strength. Several thousand research program participants have demonstrated to us that the strength-training guidelines in the Get Stronger, Feel Younger Plan provide a most sensible and successful approach for optimally building muscle and reducing fat.

Our Standard Strength-Training Program is recommended not only for people who are new to strength training but also for those who have limited time available for exercise. This basic and time-efficient training protocol provides *one* set of *one* exercise for each major muscle group and requires only 20 minutes for completion. Try to complete three workouts per week on nonconsecutive days—Monday, Wednesday, and Friday; or Tuesday, Thursday, and Saturday. If this does not fit with your schedule, you can still attain excellent results by training at least 2 days each week (for example, Monday and Thursday, or Wednesday and Saturday).

PROGRAM PROTOCOL

Every exercise repetition must be performed with proper form to maximize your training effectiveness. This requires full-range exercise movements and controlled exercise speeds. Generally, each lifting action (positive muscle contraction) should take about 2 seconds, and each lowering action (negative muscle contraction) should take about 4 seconds. Use a resistance that permits

8 to 12 properly performed repetitions. When you can complete 12 repetitions with good form in two consecutive training sessions, increase the resistance by about 5 percent for your next workout. We recommend approximately 60-second rest periods between successive exercises, which should permit program completion within 20 minutes.

Weight-Stack Machine Exercise Sequence

The following chart presents the Get Stronger, Feel Younger Standard Strength-Training Program recommended exercise sequence for fitness facility workouts using weight-stack machines. We strongly suggest that you train in this particular order, namely, from larger to smaller muscle groups and alternating opposing muscle groups. Each of the 10 weight-stack machine exercises is described and illustrated in Chapter 5.

GET STRONGER, FEEL YOUNGER STANDARD STRENGTH-TRAINING PROGRAM FOR WEIGHT-STACK MACHINES

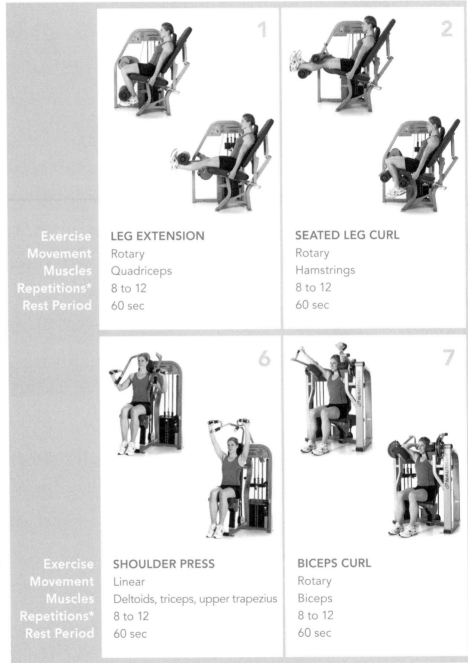

Exercise	LEG EXTENSION	SEATED LEG CURL
Movement	Rotary	Rotary
Muscles	Quadriceps	Hamstrings
Repetitions*	8 to 12	8 to 12
Rest Period	60 sec	60 sec

*When you are able to complete 12 good repetitions in two consecutive training sessions, raise the resistance by about 5 percent for your next workout.

Exercise	SHOULDER PRESS	BICEPS CURL
Movement	Linear	Rotary
Muscles	Deltoids, triceps, upper trapezius	Biceps
Repetitions*	8 to 12	8 to 12
Rest Period	60 sec	60 sec

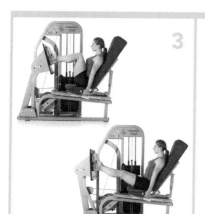

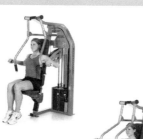

LEG PRESS
Linear
Quadriceps, hamstrings
8 to 12
60 sec

CHEST PRESS
Linear
Pectoralis major, triceps
8 to 12
60 sec

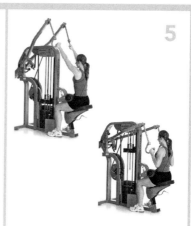

PULLDOWN
Linear
Latissimus dorsi, biceps
8 to 12
60 sec

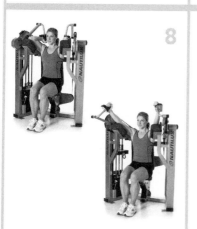

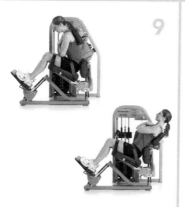

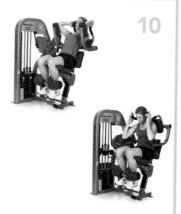

TRICEPS EXTENSION
Rotary
Triceps
8 to 12
60 sec

LOWER BACK EXTENSION
Rotary
Erector spinae
8 to 12
60 sec

ABDOMINAL CURL
Rotary
Rectus abdominis
8 to 12
60 sec

Dumbbell/Body-Weight Exercise Sequence

The following chart presents the Get Stronger, Feel Younger Standard Strength-Training Program recommended exercise sequence for home workouts using dumbbells and body-weight resistance. We strongly suggest that you train in this order, namely, from larger to smaller muscle groups and alternating opposing muscle groups. Because it is difficult to target individual leg muscles with free weights, the three leg exercises address both the quadriceps and hamstrings. By using different movement patterns and changing lead legs, each leg exercise should provide a specific muscle fatigue pattern and productive strength-building stimulus. Each of the 10 dumbbell and body-weight exercises is described and illustrated in Chapter 5.

GET STRONGER, FEEL YOUNGER STANDARD STRENGTH-TRAINING PROGRAM FOR DUMBBELLS AND BODY-WEIGHT RESISTANCE

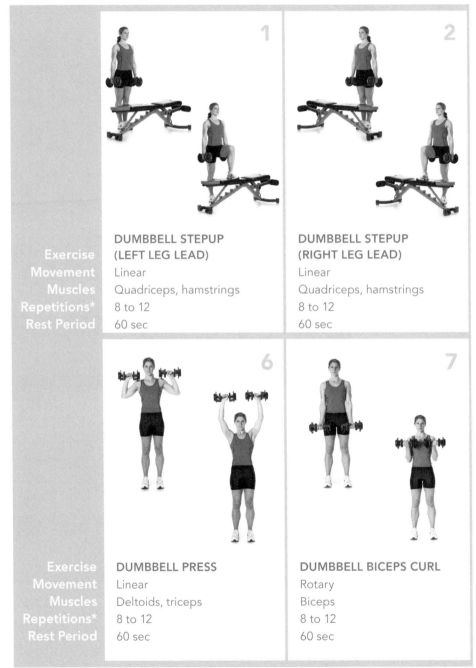

Whenever you complete 12 good repetitions in two consecutive training sessions, raise the resistance by about 5 percent for your next workout, except for body-weight exercises, which should be performed for additional repetitions.

	1	2
Exercise	DUMBBELL STEPUP (LEFT LEG LEAD)	DUMBBELL STEPUP (RIGHT LEG LEAD)
Movement	Linear	Linear
Muscles	Quadriceps, hamstrings	Quadriceps, hamstrings
Repetitions*	8 to 12	8 to 12
Rest Period	60 sec	60 sec

	6	7
Exercise	DUMBBELL PRESS	DUMBBELL BICEPS CURL
Movement	Linear	Rotary
Muscles	Deltoids, triceps	Biceps
Repetitions*	8 to 12	8 to 12
Rest Period	60 sec	60 sec

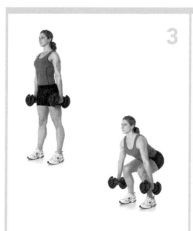

3

DUMBBELL SQUAT

Linear

Quadriceps, hamstrings

8 to 12

60 sec

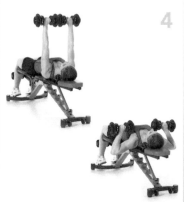

4

DUMBBELL BENCH PRESS

Linear

Pectoralis major, triceps

8 to 12

60 sec

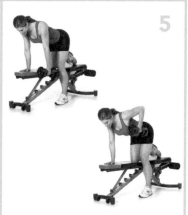

5

DUMBBELL ROW

Linear

Latissimus dorsi, biceps

8 to 12

60 sec

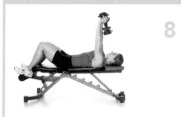

8

DUMBBELL TRICEPS EXTENSION

Rotary

Triceps

8 to 12

60 sec

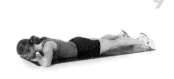
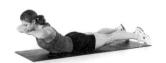

9

BODY-WEIGHT TRUNK EXTENSION

Rotary

Erector spinae

8 to 12

60 sec

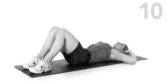
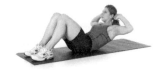

10

BODY-WEIGHT TRUNK CURL

Rotary

Rectus abdominis

8 to 12

60 sec

Bowflex Exercise Sequence

The following chart presents the Get Stronger, Feel Younger Standard Strength-Training Program recommended exercise sequence for home workouts using a Bowflex apparatus. We encourage you to train in this order, namely, from larger to smaller muscle groups and alternating opposing muscle groups. Each of the 10 Bowflex exercises is described and illustrated in Chapter 5.

GET STRONGER, FEEL YOUNGER STANDARD STRENGTH-TRAINING PROGRAM FOR BOWFLEX

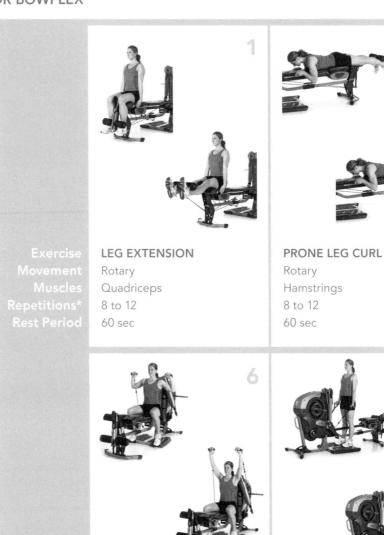

When you are able to complete 12 good repetitions in two consecutive training sessions, raise the resistance by about 5 percent for your next workout.

Exercise	LEG EXTENSION	PRONE LEG CURL
Movement	Rotary	Rotary
Muscles	Quadriceps	Hamstrings
Repetitions*	8 to 12	8 to 12
Rest Period	60 sec	60 sec

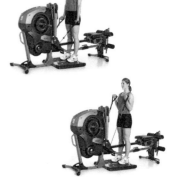

Exercise	SHOULDER PRESS	BICEPS CURL
Movement	Linear	Rotary
Muscles	Deltoids, triceps	Biceps
Repetitions*	8 to 12	8 to 12
Rest Period	60 sec	60 sec

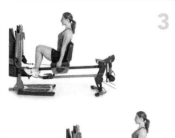

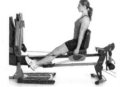

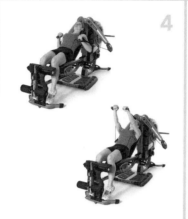

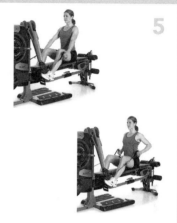

3

LEG PRESS
Linear
Quadriceps, hamstrings
8 to 12
60 sec

4

CHEST PRESS
Linear
Pectoralis major, triceps
8 to 12
60 sec

5

SEATED ROW
Linear
Latissimus dorsi, biceps
8 to 12
60 sec

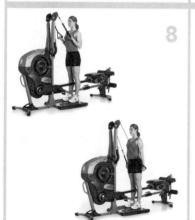

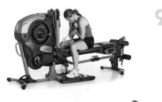

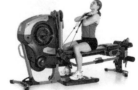

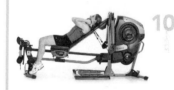

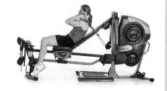

8

TRICEPS EXTENSION
Rotary
Triceps
8 to 12
60 sec

9

LOWER BACK EXTENSION
Rotary
Erector spinae
8 to 12
60 sec

10

ABDOMINAL FLEXION
Rotary
Rectus abdominis
8 to 12
60 sec

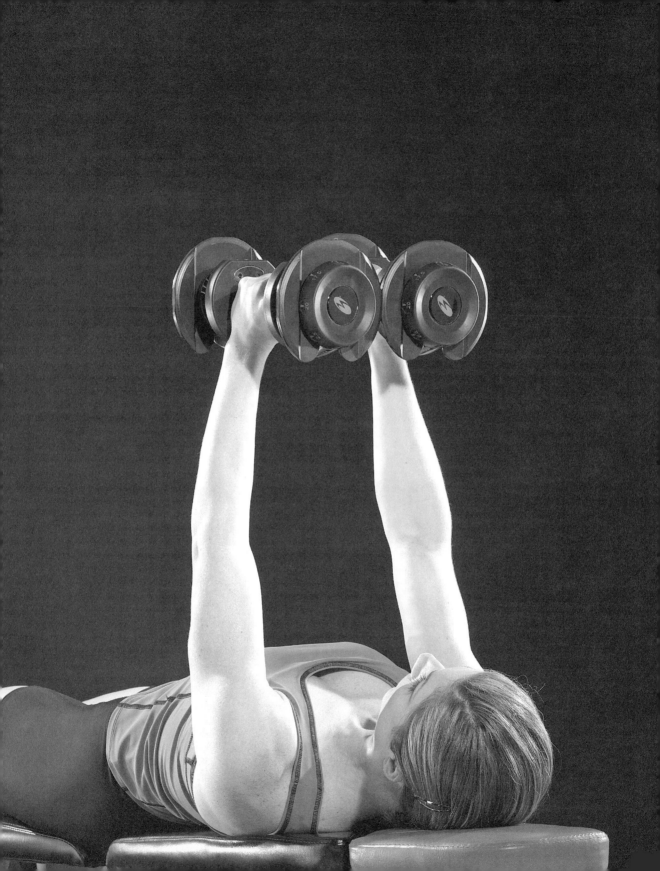

CHAPTER 8

MUSCLE-BUILDING PROGRAM FOR ADVANCED EXERCISERS

As exercisers become more advanced, they are typically advised to increase their training volume, or the amount of sets they perform, in order to make further improvement and to attain additional body composition benefits. Unfortunately, as normally applied, doubling the number of exercise sets more than doubles the total training time. This is because you must take a sufficient rest period between sets of the same exercise, and the most prevalent average rest period is about 2 minutes.

So let's assume that you take 1 minute to perform a 10-repetition exercise set, that you take a 1-minute rest between different exercises, and that you take a 2-minute rest between sets of the same exercise. If you complete one set each of 10 different exercises, your total training time is less than 20 minutes, as illustrated in the first table below:

Time for exercise performance (10 exercises × 1 set × 1 minute per set)	10 minutes
Time for rest periods between different exercises (10 exercises × 1-minute rest between exercises)	9 minutes
TOTAL TRAINING TIME	**19 MINUTES**

However, if you complete two sets of 10 different exercises, your total training time is approximately 50 minutes, as calculated below:

Time for exercise performance (10 exercises × 2 sets × 1 minute per set)	20 minutes
Time for rest periods between different exercises (10 exercises × 1-minute rest between exercises)	9 minutes
Time for rest periods between sets of the same exercise (10 exercises × 2 minutes between paired sets)	20 minutes
TOTAL TRAINING TIME	**49 MINUTES**

So how can we increase the training volume, and the muscle-building stimulus, without an unrealistic time commitment? In essence, our Advanced Strength-Training Program doubles the number of exercises for each major muscle group, and thereby doubles the number of sets performed. However, it does so in a much more effective and time-efficient way. Instead of completing two sets of the same exercise for the target muscle group, you will perform two related but different exercises for the same muscle group. This is advantageous in two ways. First, instead of providing two identical bouts of exercise (same training stimulus) to your target muscle group, you will provide two nonidentical bouts of exercise (different training stimuli) to your target muscle group for an enhanced training effect. Second, instead of resting 2 minutes between paired sets of the same exercise, you will take only 20 seconds of recovery time between two related but different exercises, for a shorter training session.

Consider the following example comparing traditional strength training with our Advanced Strength-Training Program for just one major muscle group, the quadriceps muscles of the front thighs.

TRADITIONAL QUADRICEPS WORKOUT

First exercise set (10 leg extensions)	About 1 minute
Rest period between paired exercise sets	About 2 minutes
Second exercise set (10 leg extensions)	About 1 minute
TOTAL TRAINING TIME	**ABOUT 4 MINUTES**

Result: Two identical exercise bouts for the quadriceps muscles resulting in a moderate muscle-building stimulus.

GET STRONGER, FEEL YOUNGER QUADRICEPS WORKOUT

First exercise set (10 to 12 leg extensions)	About 1 minute
Recovery time between the related but different exercises	About 20 seconds
Second exercise set (8 to 10 leg presses)	About 1 minute
TOTAL TRAINING TIME	**ABOUT 2 MINUTES AND 20 SECONDS**

Result: Two related but different exercise bouts for the quadriceps muscles resulting in a high muscle-building stimulus in approximately one-half the training time.

You may ask how you can possibly do two productive exercises for the quadriceps muscles with only a 20-second recovery period. The key to the Get Stronger, Feel Younger Advanced Strength-Training Program is to first perform a rotary-action exercise that fatigues the target muscle group, followed closely by a linear-action exercise that further fatigues the target muscle group.

Here is how it works. The initial rotary-action exercise largely isolates the target muscle group and works it to momentary failure (first-level strength stimulus). The follow-up linear-action exercise also addresses the target muscle

QUESTIONS AND ANSWERS

The basic premise behind the Get Stronger, Feel Younger Advanced Strength-Training Program is to perform a rotary exercise for the target muscle group, followed 20 seconds later by a linear exercise for the target muscle group.

Why is the first paired exercise a rotary movement?

The rotary exercise involves one joint movement that essentially singles out the target muscle group. For example, the lateral raise is a rotary exercise that specifically works the deltoid muscles of the shoulders. When performed properly, the rotary exercise effectively fatigues the target muscle group.

Why do you rest 20 seconds between the paired exercises?

First, a 20-second recovery period is long enough to replenish much of the anaerobic energy supply that was used to perform the first exercise, thereby ensuring plenty of muscle fuel for the second exercise. Second, a 20-second recovery period is *not long enough* for fatigue recovery in the force-producing fibers of the target muscles. This requires the target muscles to perform the second exercise in a prefatigued state.

Why is the second paired exercise a linear movement?

The linear exercise involves two joint movements that require about equal effort from the prefatigued target muscle group and from a *fresh assisting muscle group.* For example, the shoulder press is a linear exercise that uses both the prefatigued deltoid muscles of the shoulders and fresh triceps muscles of the arms. When performed properly, the linear exercise pushes the target muscle group to a deeper level of fatigue, thereby producing a greater muscle-building stimulus.

group with help from fresh assisting muscles and again works it to momentary failure (second-level strength stimulus).

Let's review how you would apply our Advanced Strength-Training Program to your quadriceps muscles. You first perform a set of 10 to 12 repetitions of leg extensions (rotary-action exercise) to the point of momentary muscle failure (can't complete another repetition) to fatigue your quadriceps muscles (first-level strength stimulus). You'll take a 20-second recovery period. Then you'll perform a set of 8 to 10 repetitions of leg presses (linear-action exercise) to the point of momentary muscle failure (can't complete another repetition) to further fatigue your quadriceps muscles (second-level strength stimulus). It is possible to work the quadriceps twice in close succession because the follow-up leg press exercise uses both the prefatigued quadriceps muscles and fresh hamstring muscles. While rotary-action exercises like leg extensions use one muscle group, linear-action exercises like leg presses use two or more muscle groups, only one of which is prefatigued. With help from the fresh assisting muscles, your target muscle group can be productively pushed to a deeper level of fatigue and thereby experience a more effective training stimulus.

While we do not discredit the traditional training method, we believe that our Advanced Strength-Training Program provides more muscle-building stimulus in much less time. Given our example, within a 2-minute and 20-second time period, your quadriceps muscles experience two appropriately different and high-intensity bouts of resistance exercise. From a physiological perspective, you provide your quadriceps muscles with two different movement patterns that cumulatively involve more muscle fibers than repeating the same exercise twice. From a psychological perspective, you look forward to performing two successive exercises that involve different movement actions and fatigue patterns, rather than repeating the same exercise twice.

PROGRAM PROTOCOL

We cannot emphasize enough that every exercise repetition must be performed with proper form to maximize your training effectiveness. This requires full-range exercise movements and controlled exercise speeds. Generally, each lifting action (positive muscle contraction) should take about 2 seconds, and each lowering action (negative muscle contraction) should take about 4 seconds.

The first paired exercise is a rotary movement that is meant to fatigue the target muscle group. This exercise should be performed with a resistance that you can lift between 10 and 12 repetitions. When you can complete 12 repetitions of the rotary exercise in two consecutive training sessions, the resistance should be increased by approximately 5 percent for your next workout.

The second paired exercise is a linear movement that is designed to further fatigue the target muscle group with assistance from a fresh muscle group. This exercise should be performed with a resistance that you can lift between 8 and 10 repetitions. When you can complete 10 repetitions of the linear exercise in two consecutive training sessions, the resistance should be increased by about 5 percent for your next training session.

Rest no more than 20 seconds between the first and second paired exercise for each target muscle group. We recommend approximately 60-second rest periods between exercises for different muscle groups, which should permit program completion in about 40 minutes. Begin training three nonconsecutive days per week, such as Mondays, Wednesdays, and Fridays or Tuesdays, Thursdays, and Saturdays. If your muscles do not fully recover between these high-intensity workouts, cut back to two training sessions a week, such as Mondays and Thursdays or Wednesdays and Saturdays.

Weight-Stack Machine Exercise Sequence

The following chart presents the Get Stronger, Feel Younger Advanced Strength-Training Program recommended exercise sequence for fitness facility workouts using weight-stack machines. You will note that the first 14 exercises involve prefatigue training for the major muscles of the legs, upper body, and arms. The final four exercises cumulatively work all of the core muscle groups in the midsection area of the body. We strongly suggest that you train in this order, namely, from larger to smaller muscle groups, alternating opposing muscle groups, and concluding each workout with the four-exercise series for your core (midsection) muscles. Each of the 18 weight-stack machine exercises is described and illustrated in Chapter 5.

GET STRONGER, FEEL YOUNGER ADVANCED STRENGTH-TRAINING PROGRAM FOR WEIGHT-STACK MACHINES

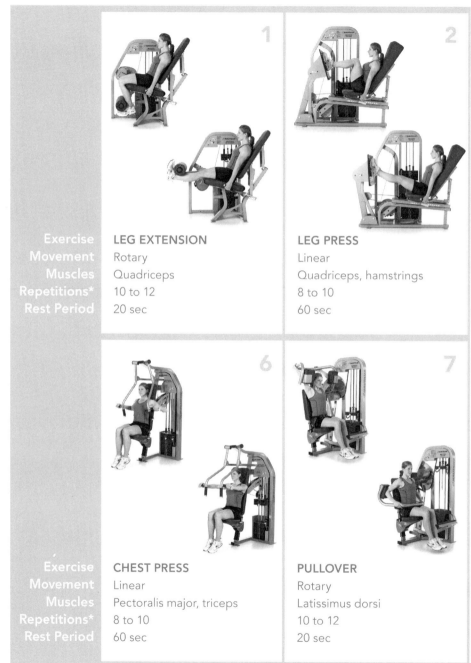

Whenever you complete 12 good repetitions of the rotary exercises twice in a row, raise the resistance by about 5 percent for your next workout. Whenever you complete 10 good repetitions of the linear exercises twice in a row, raise the resistance by about 5 percent for your next workout.

Exercise	**LEG EXTENSION**	**LEG PRESS**
Movement	Rotary	Linear
Muscles	Quadriceps	Quadriceps, hamstrings
Repetitions*	10 to 12	8 to 10
Rest Period	20 sec	60 sec

Exercise	**CHEST PRESS**	**PULLOVER**
Movement	Linear	Rotary
Muscles	Pectoralis major, triceps	Latissimus dorsi
Repetitions*	8 to 10	10 to 12
Rest Period	60 sec	20 sec

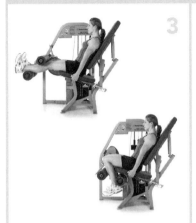

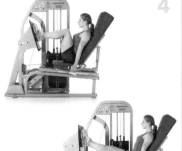

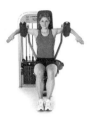

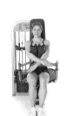

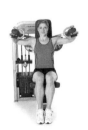

SEATED LEG CURL
Rotary
Hamstrings
10 to 12
20 sec

LEG PRESS
Linear
Hamstrings, quadriceps
8 to 10
60 sec

CHEST CROSS
Rotary
Pectoralis major
10 to 12
20 sec

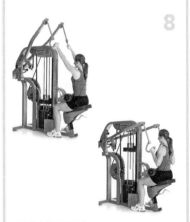

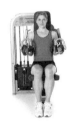

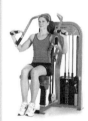

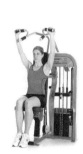

PULLDOWN
Linear
Latissimus dorsi, biceps
8 to 10
60 sec

LATERAL RAISE
Rotary
Deltoids
10 to 12
20 sec

SHOULDER PRESS
Linear
Deltoids, triceps
8 to 10
60 sec

(continued)

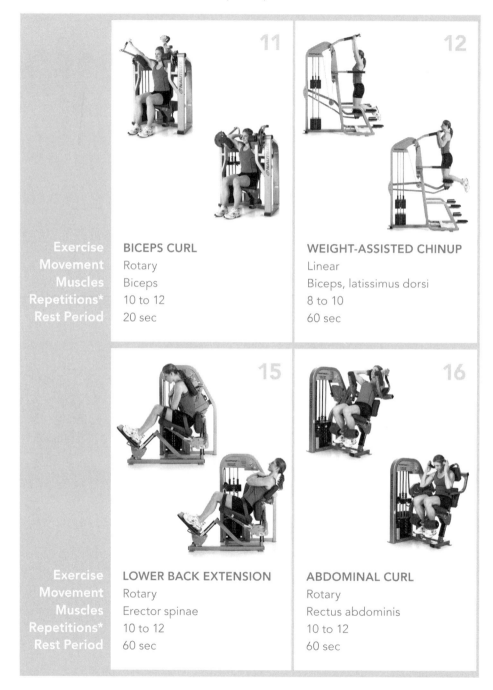

	11 BICEPS CURL	12 WEIGHT-ASSISTED CHINUP
Exercise	BICEPS CURL	WEIGHT-ASSISTED CHINUP
Movement	Rotary	Linear
Muscles	Biceps	Biceps, latissimus dorsi
Repetitions*	10 to 12	8 to 10
Rest Period	20 sec	60 sec

	15 LOWER BACK EXTENSION	16 ABDOMINAL CURL
Exercise	LOWER BACK EXTENSION	ABDOMINAL CURL
Movement	Rotary	Rotary
Muscles	Erector spinae	Rectus abdominis
Repetitions*	10 to 12	10 to 12
Rest Period	60 sec	60 sec

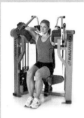
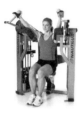

13

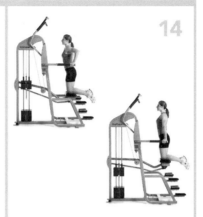

14

TRICEPS EXTENSION
Rotary
Triceps
10 to 12
20 sec

WEIGHT-ASSISTED BAR DIP
Linear
Triceps, pectoralis major
8 to 10
60 sec

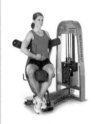
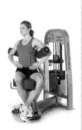

17

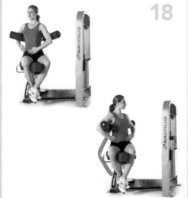

18

ROTARY TORSO (CLOCKWISE)
Rotary
Left external, right internal
  obliques
10 to 12
60 sec

ROTARY TORSO
(COUNTERCLOCKWISE)
Rotary
Right external, left internal obliques
10 to 12
60 sec

Dumbbell/Band/Body-Weight Exercise Sequence

The following chart presents the Get Stronger, Feel Younger Advanced Strength-Training Program recommended exercise sequence for home workouts using dumbbells, bands, and body-weight resistance. You will note that the first 14 exercises involve prefatigue training for the major muscles of the legs, upper body, and arms. The final four exercises cumulatively work all of the core muscle groups in the midsection area of the body. We strongly suggest that you train in this order, namely, from larger to smaller muscle groups and alternating opposing muscle groups, and concluding each workout with the four-exercise series for your core (midsection) muscles. Because it is difficult to target individual leg muscles with free weights, the four leg exercises address both the quadriceps and hamstrings. By using different movement patterns and changing lead legs, each leg exercise should provide a specific muscle fatigue pattern and productive strength-building stimulus. Each of the 18 dumbbell, band, and body-weight exercises is described and illustrated in Chapter 5.

GET STRONGER, FEEL YOUNGER ADVANCED STRENGTH-TRAINING PROGRAM FOR DUMBBELL, BAND, AND BODY-WEIGHT RESISTANCE

Whenever you complete 12 good repetitions of the rotary exercises twice in a row, raise the resistance by about 5 percent for your next workout, except for the body-weight exercises, which should be performed for additional repetitions. Whenever you complete 10 good repetitions of the linear exercises twice in a row, raise the resistance by about 5 percent for your next workout.

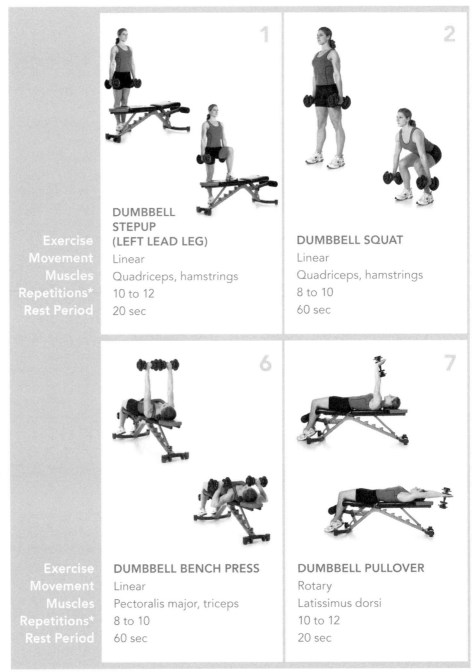

Exercise	**DUMBBELL STEPUP (LEFT LEAD LEG)**	**DUMBBELL SQUAT**
Movement	Linear	Linear
Muscles	Quadriceps, hamstrings	Quadriceps, hamstrings
Repetitions*	10 to 12	8 to 10
Rest Period	20 sec	60 sec

Exercise	**DUMBBELL BENCH PRESS**	**DUMBBELL PULLOVER**
Movement	Linear	Rotary
Muscles	Pectoralis major, triceps	Latissimus dorsi
Repetitions*	8 to 10	10 to 12
Rest Period	60 sec	20 sec

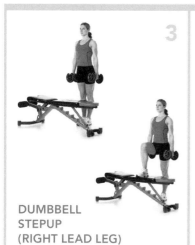

**DUMBBELL
STEPUP
(RIGHT LEAD LEG)**
Linear
Quadriceps, hamstrings
10 to 12
20 sec

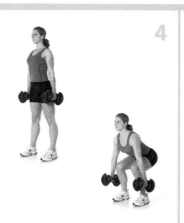

DUMBBELL SQUAT
Linear
Quadriceps, hamstrings
8 to 10
60 sec

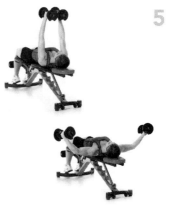

DUMBBELL FLY
Rotary
Pectoralis major
10 to 12
20 sec

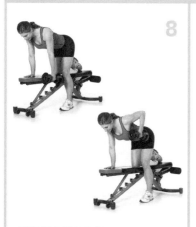

DUMBBELL ROW
Linear
Latissimus dorsi, biceps
8 to 10
60 sec

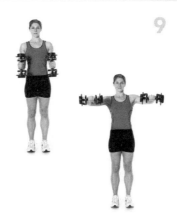

DUMBBELL LATERAL RAISE
Rotary
Deltoids
10 to 12
20 sec

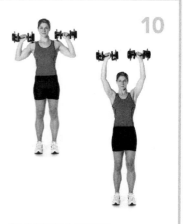

DUMBBELL PRESS
Linear
Deltoids, triceps
8 to 10
60 sec

(continued)

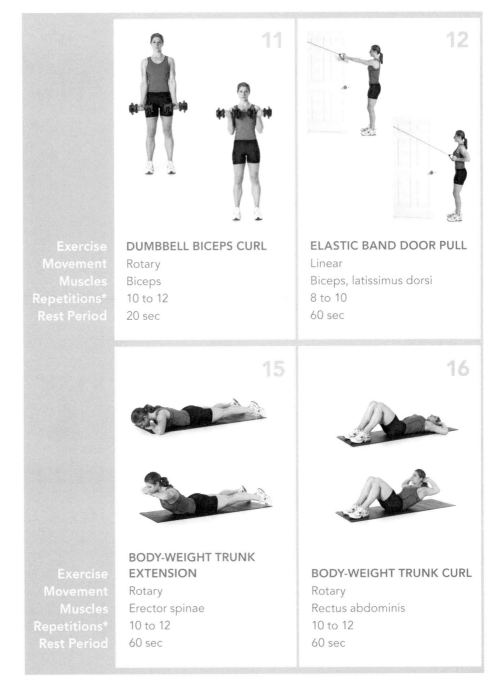

	11	12
	DUMBBELL BICEPS CURL	**ELASTIC BAND DOOR PULL**
Exercise		
Movement	Rotary	Linear
Muscles	Biceps	Biceps, latissimus dorsi
Repetitions*	10 to 12	8 to 10
Rest Period	20 sec	60 sec

	15	16
	BODY-WEIGHT TRUNK EXTENSION	**BODY-WEIGHT TRUNK CURL**
Exercise		
Movement	Rotary	Rotary
Muscles	Erector spinae	Rectus abdominis
Repetitions*	10 to 12	10 to 12
Rest Period	60 sec	60 sec

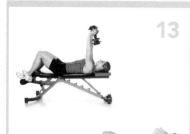

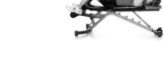

13

DUMBBELL TRICEPS EXTENSION

Rotary

Triceps

10 to 12

20 sec

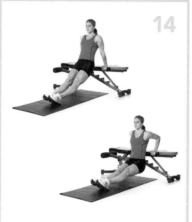

14

BODY-WEIGHT BENCH DIP

Linear

Triceps, pectoralis major

8 to 10

60 sec

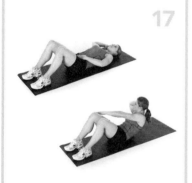

17

BODY-WEIGHT TRUNK CURL (ROTATION CLOCKWISE)

Rotary

Left external obliques, right
  internal obliques, rectus
  abdominis

10 to 12

60 sec

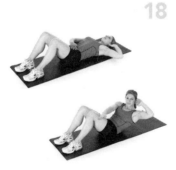

18

BODY-WEIGHT TRUNK CURL (ROTATION COUNTER-CLOCKWISE)

Rotary

Right external obliques, left
  internal obliques, rectus
  abdominis

10 to 12

60 sec

Bowflex and Body-Weight Exercise Sequence

The following chart presents the Get Stronger, Feel Younger Advanced Strength-Training Program recommended exercise sequence for home workouts using a Bowflex apparatus and body-weight resistance. You will note that the first 14 exercises involve prefatigue training for the major muscles of the legs, upper body, and arms. The final four exercises cumulatively work all of the core muscle groups in the midsection area of the body. We encourage you to train in this order, namely from larger to smaller muscle groups, alternating opposing muscle groups, and concluding each workout with the four-exercise series for your core (midsection) muscles. Each of the 18 Bowflex and body-weight exercises is described and illustrated in Chapter 5.

GET STRONGER, FEEL YOUNGER ADVANCED STRENGTH-TRAINING PROGRAM FOR BOWFLEX AND BODY-WEIGHT RESISTANCE

*Whenever you complete 12 good repetitions of the rotary exercises twice in a row, raise the resistance by about 5 percent for your next workout, except for the body-weight exercises, which should be performed for additional repetitions. Whenever you complete 10 good repetitions of the linear exercises twice in a row, raise the resistance by about 5 percent for your next workout.

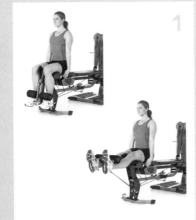

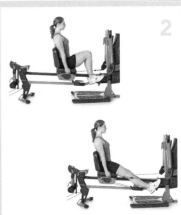

Exercise	**LEG EXTENSION**	**LEG PRESS**
Movement	Rotary	Linear
Muscles	Quadriceps	Quadriceps, hamstrings
Repetitions*	10 to 12	8 to 10
Rest Period	20 sec	60 sec

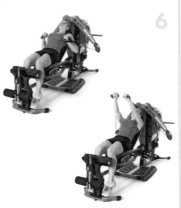

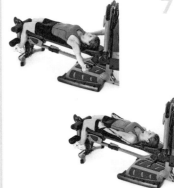

Exercise	**CHEST PRESS**	**LATERAL FLY**
Movement	Linear	Rotary
Muscles	Pectoralis major, triceps	Latissimus dorsi
Repetitions*	8 to 10	10 to 12
Rest Period	60 sec	20 sec

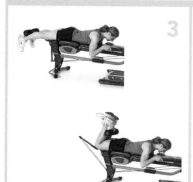

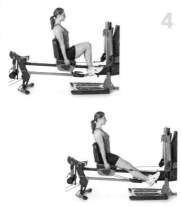

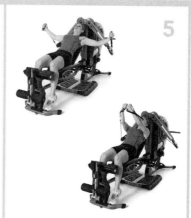

PRONE LEG CURL
Rotary
Hamstrings
10 to 12
20 sec

LEG PRESS
Linear
Quadriceps, hamstrings
8 to 10
60 sec

CHEST CROSS
Rotary
Pectoralis major
10 to 12
20 sec

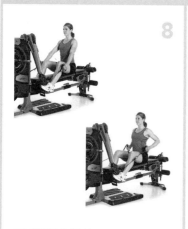

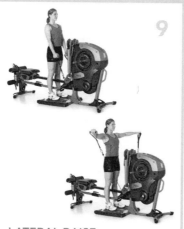

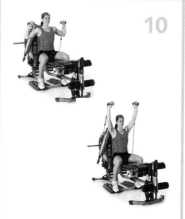

SEATED ROW
Linear
Latissimus dorsi, biceps
8 to 10
60 sec

LATERAL RAISE
Rotary
Deltoids
10 to 12
20 sec

SHOULDER PRESS
Linear
Deltoids, triceps
8 to 10
60 sec

(continued)

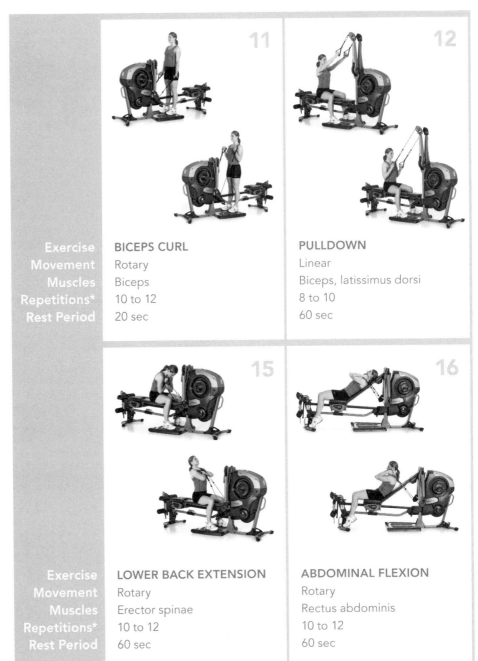

	11 BICEPS CURL	**12 PULLDOWN**
Exercise	BICEPS CURL	PULLDOWN
Movement	Rotary	Linear
Muscles	Biceps	Biceps, latissimus dorsi
Repetitions*	10 to 12	8 to 10
Rest Period	20 sec	60 sec

	15 LOWER BACK EXTENSION	**16 ABDOMINAL FLEXION**
Exercise	LOWER BACK EXTENSION	ABDOMINAL FLEXION
Movement	Rotary	Rotary
Muscles	Erector spinae	Rectus abdominis
Repetitions*	10 to 12	10 to 12
Rest Period	60 sec	60 sec

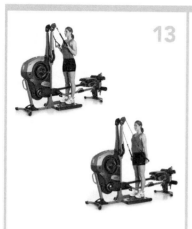

13

TRICEPS EXTENSION
Rotary
Triceps
10 to 12
20 sec

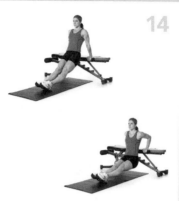

14

BODY-WEIGHT BENCH DIP
Linear
Triceps, pectoralis major
8 to 10
60 sec

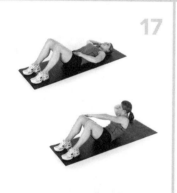

17

BODY-WEIGHT TRUNK CURL (ROTATION CLOCKWISE)
Rotary
Left external obliques, right
  internal obliques, rectus
  abdominis
10 to 12
60 sec

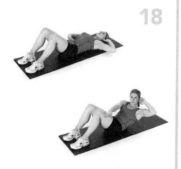

18

BODY-WEIGHT TRUNK CURL (ROTATION COUNTER-CLOCKWISE)
Rotary
Right external obliques, left
  internal obliques, rectus
  abdominis
10 to 12
60 sec

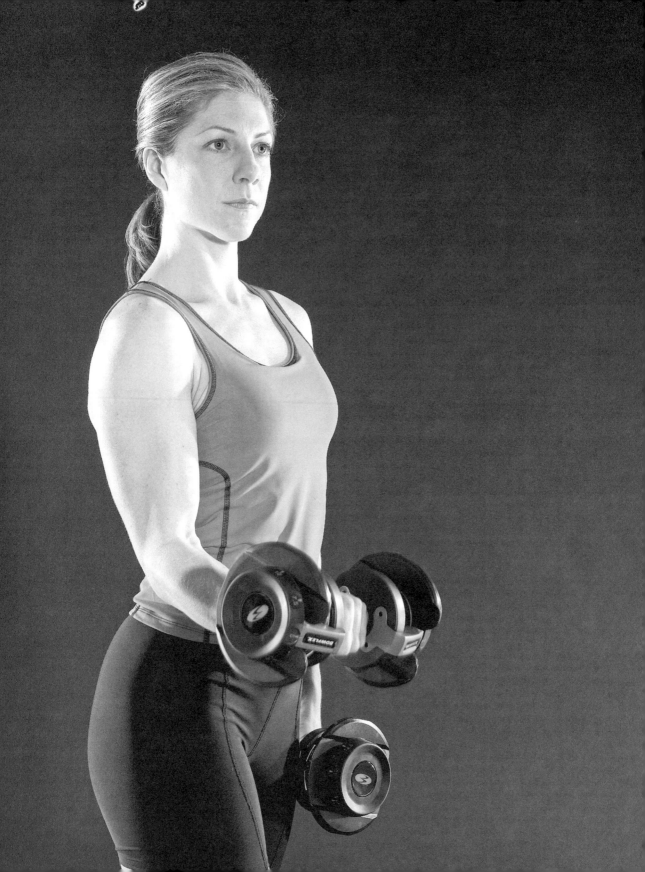

CHAPTER 9

HOW DO I MEASURE SUCCESS?

Most people who begin a diet program associate success with lower body weight. They live and die by the bathroom scale, which is most unfortunate. Scales tell you how much a package weighs, so to speak, but not what is in the package. The package we call our body consists of two major components, referred to as fat weight and lean weight (muscles, bones, blood, organs, and so forth). A woman who is 40 percent fat is unhealthy from a body composition perspective, regardless of her body weight. On the other hand, a woman who is 20 percent fat is very healthy from a body composition perspective, whether she weighs 120 pounds or 160 pounds.

While a bathroom scale may give you a general picture of your body weight, a full-length mirror will give you a much better view of your physical condition and personal appearance. Body measurements may also be helpful in this regard. For example, let's say a woman following the Get Stronger, Feel Younger

Plan loses only 4 pounds according to the bathroom scale. However, her thigh measurement decreases by 1 inch, and her waist measurement decreases by 3 inches. How can this be with such a small weight loss? A body composition assessment reveals that she has added 4 pounds of muscle and lost 8 pounds of fat. On the scale, this shows up as a 4-pound weight loss, but she has actually achieved a 12-pound improvement in her body composition, physical fitness, and personal appearance, as evidenced also by her better body measurements.

One of the reasons we recommend that you begin your muscle-building program at a YMCA, health club, or other fitness facility is to receive periodic body composition analyses. Fitness professionals can accurately evaluate your body composition in a matter of minutes, thereby telling you what percentage of your body weight is fat and what percentage is lean tissue. Reassessments will reveal how much fat you have lost and how much muscle you have added as a result of your strength-training program.

BODY COMPOSITION

Body composition success is consistent with lower percent body fat readings. Although beauty is in the eye of the beholder, ideal body composition ranges for women are 20 to 24 percent fat, and ideal body composition ranges for men are 12 to 16 percent fat. While you may prefer to be slightly above or below these recommended percent fat ranges, they certainly represent good goals and excellent measures of success. Don't worry about body weight. If your body composition is healthy, then your body weight is right for you. Don't even look at standard height and weight charts because they do not account for muscle development and seriously underestimate ideal body weights for strength-trained men and women.

Most YMCAs and fitness centers can assess your body composition (percent fat) quickly and easily by means of skinfold calipers, electrical impedance, or similar techniques. These important assessments should be performed by qualified fitness professionals before you begin the Get Stronger, Feel Younger Plan and every 10 weeks thereafter to check your progress and to reinforce your exercise efforts.

RESTING METABOLIC RATE

So your first measure of success, other than looking better, feeling better, fitting into your clothes better, and functioning better, is improved body composition. A related measure of success is a higher resting metabolism, which can also be assessed at some YMCAs and fitness centers. Remember that more muscle is similar to more cylinders in your automobile engine. Also, more muscle enables you to use more energy (calories) all day long (24 hours a day). After 10 weeks of strength training, you should add about 3 pounds of muscle, and your resting metabolic rate should increase by about 7 percent (approximately 100 calories per day). Other things remaining the same, your higher metabolism could result in a fat loss of almost 1 pound per month. Checking your resting metabolism periodically throughout the Get Stronger, Feel Younger Plan will reveal how much more energy you are using daily and how you are transitioning from a small-engine, low-power body to a large-engine, high-power body that burns lots of energy and looks more like a sports car.

MUSCLE STRENGTH

Muscle strength is the most basic measure of physical fitness. Every movement you make uses a certain percentage of your maximum muscle strength. Because we live in such a modernized and mechanized society, we seldom recognize the importance of a strong and functional musculoskeletal system. But strong muscles play a major role in many sports, recreational, and work activities. They also help protect you against a variety of injuries and degenerative diseases.

We believe that muscle strength is both an admirable objective in itself and a means to numerous ends related to health, fitness, and functionality. Muscle strength is easy to assess, even without determining the heaviest resistance that you can lift one time. Most people can complete 10 repetitions with 75 percent of their maximum resistance. So, if you are presently doing 10 shoulder presses with 75 pounds, your maximum strength in this exercise should be approximately 100 pounds.

However, because there is a direct relationship between the resistance you can lift 10 times and the resistance you can lift once, the simplest way to assess your strength improvement is by the progressive increases in your exercise weight loads. If your shoulder press performance (one set of 10 repetitions) increases from 75 pounds to 100 pounds, then you have experienced a 33 percent strength gain in your shoulder muscles (25 lb/75 lb = 33% strength improvement). You may evaluate your strength development on all of your training exercises simply by reviewing your workout card. For practical purposes, the leg press, chest press, pulldown, and shoulder press are typically assessed as measures of overall muscle strength. As a general guideline, you should increase your exercise weight loads 20 to 40 percent in these four major muscle exercises after just 10 weeks of training with our plan.

BONE DENSITY

Muscle tissue and bone tissue work together. That is, muscle loss is associated with bone loss, and muscle gain is associated with bone gain. As you increase your muscle mass, you should likewise increase your bone mineral density to accommodate the added muscle weight and force. This produces a stronger musculoskeletal system and reduces your risk of osteoporosis and related functional complications. Strength training also benefits the tendons, ligaments, and connective tissues that protect your joint structures and lessens the chances of experiencing problems associated with tendonitis, arthritis, lower back pain, and similar debilitating conditions.

Although bone mineral density is not typically assessed at fitness centers, you can schedule a convenient appointment at most medical facilities. Various studies indicate that bone mineral density increases between 1 and 12 percent after several months of strength training depending on your age, gender, and other factors such as nutrient intake.

BLOOD PRESSURE

While you should certainly have your physician's approval prior to participating in any exercise program, research reveals that sensible strength training is actually beneficial with respect to high blood pressure. Our studies show that your blood pressure readings will most likely be temporarily lower following your strength-training session than before you started. And based on our research with several hundred subjects, your resting blood pressure should be permanently lower following 10 weeks of the Get Stronger, Feel Younger Plan. On average, our participants' systolic blood pressure readings decreased by 4 mmHg, and their diastolic blood pressure readings dropped by 2 mmHg.

Many other studies confirm that properly performed strength training can produce the same beneficial effects on resting blood pressure as endurance exercise, such as walking, jogging, and cycling. Just be sure to train correctly and breathe continuously throughout every exercise set. Most YMCA and fitness center instructors are trained to accurately measure your resting blood pressure, which should be taken periodically throughout your participation in the Get Stronger, Feel Younger Plan.

BLOOD CHOLESTEROL

Strength training has been shown to improve blood lipid profiles, by both lowering the bad (LDL) cholesterol and raising the good (HDL) cholesterol. In fact, muscle-building exercise may be as effective as aerobic activity for eliciting

GET STRONGER, FEEL YOUNGER SUCCESS STORY

Marika Sanchez suffered a head and leg injury. To make matters worse, she was told that it would be impossible to return to a normal lifestyle because of its severity. "Well, as one can imagine, I became overweight, unhealthy, and depressed," says Marika, "but through my faith and the strength-training program at the South Shore YMCA, I was able to achieve what I was previously told to be impossible."

She is now in the best shape of her life. Over 6 months, her body weight decreased by more than 50 pounds, and her cholesterol decreased by almost 100 points. "At my last physical, my doctor said, 'If all my patients were like you, I'd be out of a job. Keep up the good work.' Imagine that! I have great expectations for the future."

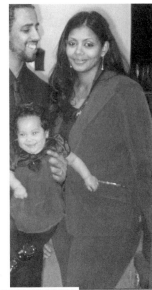

Before ▶

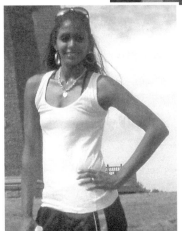

After ▶

these beneficial changes in blood cholesterol levels. Although few fitness facilities perform blood lipid assessments, you may want to ask your personal physician to check your blood cholesterol after completing the Get Stronger, Feel Younger Plan to compare with previous numbers. Better blood lipid profiles and lower blood pressure readings reduce your risk of cardiovascular diseases and stroke, which are additional benefits of regular strength training.

BLOOD GLUCOSE

If you have high blood glucose levels, following our plan should be particularly helpful. Research with prediabetic patients showed almost 25 percent better glucose utilization after 16 weeks of regular strength training, thereby reducing their risk of developing type 2 diabetes. Apparently, strength-trained muscles enhance glucose uptake from the blood, which lessens the likelihood of diabetic conditions. Blood glucose levels are typically assessed by your physician during annual medical examinations.

DIGESTIVE PROCESSES

The rate at which food passes through your gastrointestinal system is referred to as transit speed. Slow transit speeds are associated with a higher risk of colon cancer and are therefore undesirable. Research has demonstrated a 55 percent increase in gastrointestinal transit speed following 3 months of regular strength training. Faster food transit times provide many benefits, including a lower risk of illness related to the colon. If you presently experience slow gastrointestinal transit, you may be pleasantly surprised by faster food movements and more regularity following several weeks of muscle-building exercise.

BACK PAIN AND ARTHRITIS

Without question, more people have experienced lower back pain and arthritic discomfort than most other physical ailments combined. Fortunately, both of these pervasive problems respond positively to appropriate strength training. Proper performance of the lower back extension exercise reduced or eliminated lower back pain in 80 percent of the patients in a University of Florida College of Medicine study. Tufts University research revealed that muscle-building exercise concurrently increased joint function and decreased joint discomfort in arthritic patients. Keep in mind that stronger muscles function as better shock absorbers and, as such, provide important protection for your joint structures.

While not everyone who suffers from back pain or arthritis is helped by strength exercise, the results of the University of Florida and Tufts studies are certainly encouraging. If you have lower back pain or arthritis, we suggest that you first consult with your physician, then work with a qualified fitness instructor who can modify your muscle-building program accordingly. While you may not notice dramatic improvements immediately, after several weeks of sensible strength training, you should have less discomfort and more functional ability.

RECORD KEEPING

You probably didn't realize that muscle-building exercise provided so many health-related benefits. The first step for attaining these desirable strength-training outcomes is exercise consistency. Basically, if you don't train, you don't gain. The key to adding muscle, losing fat, reducing your resting blood pressure, increasing your metabolic rate, and experiencing the other physiological benefits of your strength training is keeping a regular training schedule. By all means, record each exercise session in an exercise log similar to the example shown on the opposite page. This enables you to monitor your progress, which reinforces your training efforts and reduces your chances of skipping workouts. Use one sheet for each exercise session, and make additional copies whenever necessary.

To help you with your training records, we have also included sample training log pages—complete with exercise logs—in the Appendix.

GET STRONGER, FEEL YOUNGER EXERCISE LOG

Day _____ Date _____ Time _____

EXERCISE	RESISTANCE	REPETITIONS	COMMENTS
1			
2			
3			
4			
5			
6			
7			
8			
9			
10			
11			
12			
13			
14			
15			
16			
17			
18			

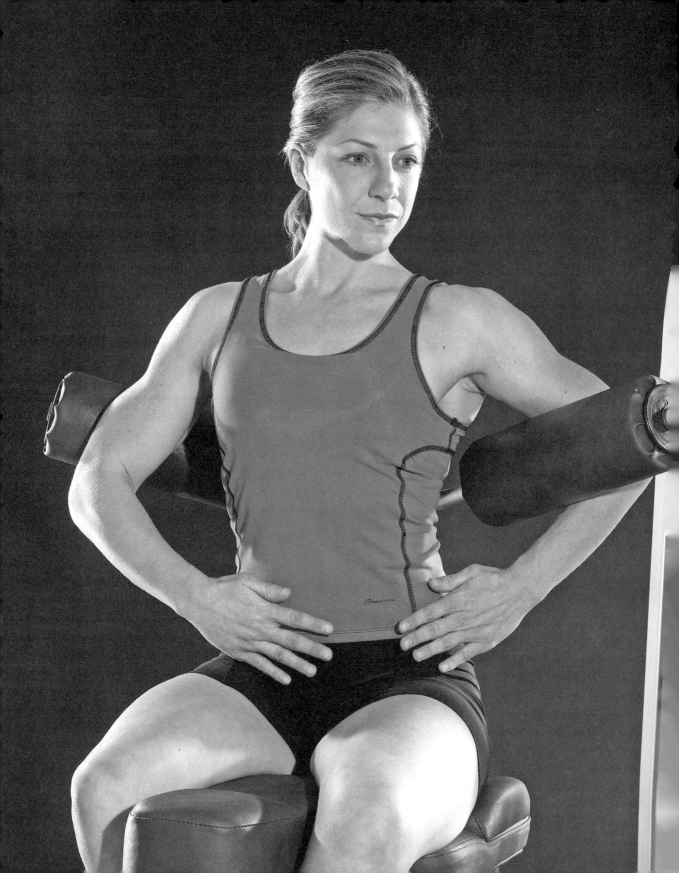

CHAPTER 10

WHAT ABOUT FOOD AND NUTRITION?

As you are now aware, the Get Stronger, Feel Younger Plan is not about "food diets," but rather a "diet" of sensible muscle-building exercise that burns calories during your workout, after your training session, and all day long as a result of a higher metabolic rate. We believe that muscle-building exercise is absolutely the most effective means for attaining and maintaining your desirable body weight and body composition. We think that this is the best approach to looking better, feeling better, and functioning better. Our plan is a proactive exercise protocol designed to improve your health, fitness, and personal appearance. This program represents a qualitative experience that *adds* something good (productive physical exercise) to your lifestyle. In contrast, a food diet typically represents a quantitative experience that *subtracts* something good (food) from your lifestyle.

Research reveals that only 50 percent of the people who begin a food diet complete the program. Even more discouraging, of those who do complete the diet program, 95 percent regain all the weight they lost during the following year. If calorie-restricted diets really worked, then the United States should have a drastically decreasing rate of obesity, because one of every two Americans is presently dieting. Unfortunately, we are experiencing the exact opposite situation, with an ever-increasing percentage of Americans classified as overweight and obese.

It is therefore rather obvious that calorie-restricted diets rarely produce permanent reductions in body weight. In fact, reduced-calorie diets are almost always more harmful than helpful, because they result in muscle loss and metabolic rate reduction. Up to 25 percent of the weight lost on typical diet programs may come from lean (muscle) tissue. For example, a 20-pound weight loss resulting from typical calorie restriction methods may actually represent a 15-pound fat loss and a 5-pound muscle loss. This undesirable outcome could reduce your resting metabolic rate by up to 10 percent, which means you must eat even less food to attain and maintain your desired body weight. Of course, this procedure is clearly self-defeating and explains why most dieters experience only short-term benefits (and long-term consequences) from popular food-restriction regimens.

Although we do not advocate most diet plans, especially those that require really low calorie counts, we do have some suggestions for sensible eating to complement the strength exercises in the Get Stronger, Feel Younger Plan. Let's begin with the premise that food is essential for living and that appropriate food selections are necessary for optimum health. For example, eating too little protein or calcium may result in a weak musculoskeletal system. Eating too little iron may lead to anemia, and insufficient dietary fiber may adversely affect gastrointestinal function. On the other hand, high fat consumption increases the risk of diabetes, heart disease, and certain types of cancer. Consuming too much salt (or too many high-sodium foods) may contribute to hypertension in some individuals.

Some people try to compensate for poor food choices by taking various nutritional supplements, but we do not support this strategy. We strongly recommend a sensible eating plan that includes a variety of vegetables, fruits, and whole grains to obtain the vitamins, minerals, antioxidants, and fiber we need for enhanced health and disease resistance.

While one author is a longtime vegan, and the other is the son of meat-eating dairy farmers, we both agree that the MyPyramid eating plan recommended by the U.S. Department of Agriculture is an excellent model for food selections and serving sizes. The MyPyramid eating plan is relatively high in carbohydrates, moderate in proteins, low in fats, and provides the following sensible guidelines for healthy eating. The table on page 154 offers examples of various foods that comprise the prescribed food categories (grains, fruits, vegetables, meats/beans, dairy), as well as suggested serving sizes to attain the recommended amounts.

WATER

Although not strictly considered a food because it contains no calories, water is certainly the most important nutrient. Keep in mind that muscle tissue is more than 75 percent water. In addition to the health benefits associated with good hydration, drinking cold water burns calories as the body conducts a warming process to get the water to body temperature. For example, ½ gallon of refrigerated water requires more than 60 calories to reach body temperature of 98.6°F. We support the standard guideline of eight glasses of water on a daily basis, and even more on exercise days. You may substitute nonalcoholic and noncaffeinated beverages such as low-fat milk, orange juice, apple juice, and grape juice for water. Although these nutritious and delicious beverages contain a considerable number of calories, they are mostly water and definitely contribute to daily hydration. Mixing juices in a 50/50 combination with carbonated water reduces the calories per glass and makes a most refreshing drink.

MYPYRAMID PLAN SAMPLE FOODS AND SUGGESTED SERVING SIZES

FOOD EXAMPLE / ONE-SERVING SIZE	FOOD EXAMPLE / ONE-SERVING SIZE
GRAINS (GET 6 OZ EVERY DAY)	
Nugget cereals, ¼ cup	Tortilla, 1
Cooked cereals, ½ cup	Rice, ⅓ cup
Flaked cereals, ¾ cup	Pasta, ½ cup
Bagel, ½	Crackers, 4
Bread, 1 slice	
FRUITS (GET 1½ CUPS EVERY DAY)	
Raisins, 2 Tbsp	Banana, 1
Dates, 3	Peach, 1
Prunes, 3	Pear, 1
Grapes, ½ cup	Melon, ¼
Berries, ¾ cup	Grapefruit, ½
Apple, 1	Pineapple, ¾ cup
VEGETABLES (GET 2½ CUPS EVERY DAY)	
Beans, ½ cup	Carrots, ½ cup
Peas, ½ cup	Tomatoes, ½ cup
Corn, ½ cup	Potatoes, ½ cup
Spinach, ½ cup	Broccoli, ½ cup
Squash, ½ cup	Cauliflower, ½ cup
MEAT AND BEANS (GET 5 OZ EVERY DAY)	
Fish, 3 oz	Dry beans, ¼ cup
Poultry, 3 oz	Canned tuna, ¼ cup
Beef, 3 oz	Tofu, ¼ cup
Egg, 1	Peanut butter, 1 Tbsp

FOOD EXAMPLE / ONE-SERVING SIZE	FOOD EXAMPLE / ONE-SERVING SIZE
DAIRY (GET 3 CUPS EVERY DAY)	
1% milk, 1 cup	Ricotta cheese, ¼ cup
Low-fat yogurt, 1 cup	Parmesan cheese, ¼ cup
Low-fat cheese, 1 oz	Fat-free evaporated milk, ½ cup
Low-fat cottage cheese, ¼ cup	
OILS (USE SPARINGLY)	
Butter, 1 tsp	Salad dressing, 1 Tbsp
Mayonnaise, 1 tsp	Sour cream, 2 Tbsp
Vegetable oil, 1 tsp	Cream cheese, 1 Tbsp

CALORIES

Losing fat is basically a matter of calories in versus calories out. If the number of calories you eat is less than the number of calories you burn, then you lose fat, which is most likely one of your main goals. However, if the calorie deficit is too large, you will also lose muscle, which should not be one of your goals. Three simple ways to sensibly reduce the number of calories you eat, without starving yourself and without sacrificing muscle, are *better food selection*, *substitution*, and *preparation*. Because fats contain twice as many calories per gram as carbohydrates and proteins, *select* foods that have less fat content. For example, fish is about 10 percent fat, white poultry meat is about 20 percent fat, dark poultry meat is about 40 percent fat, and beef is about 60 percent fat. Likewise, low-fat dairy products have significantly fewer calories than whole-milk varieties.

If you are willing to experiment, you may find that fat-free plain yogurt is an excellent lower-calorie *substitute* for sour cream on baked potatoes and for mayonnaise in potato salad. Similarly, you may learn to like lemon juice or vinegar just as much as high-calorie salad dressings.

With respect to food *preparation*, you may be surprised to learn that frying can double the calorie content of some foods due to oil absorption. We recommend baking, broiling, or microwaving as healthy alternatives to frying. We also advise against fried fast foods and those cooked in oil, such as french fries.

Although the emphasis of this book is burning calories by building larger and stronger muscles, we have included some sample meal plans for eating 2,800, 2,200, or 1,600 calories a day at the end of this chapter for those who want menu guidelines. Our exercise program participants have used these menu examples for the past several years with excellent results. Those who have closely followed the sample meal plans have actually lost twice as much fat as those who did not change their eating habits. So, if you desire a faster rate of fat loss, you may complement the strength exercises in the Get Stronger, Feel Younger Plan with the sample menu plans. Feel free to make equivalent substitutions, such as ½ cup of peas for ½ cup of green beans, 1 pear for 1 peach, 1 cup of oat flakes for 1 cup of cornflakes, 1 glass of orange juice for 1 glass of apple juice, or 3 ounces of white chicken for 3 ounces of white turkey. However, be careful not to make any *major* changes in the recommended meals because this almost always produces less program compliance and typically leads to less-successful fat loss. For example, don't substitute a dish of ice cream for a low-fat yogurt by rationalizing that they are both dairy products that help meet your calcium requirements.

EATING TO ENHANCE YOUR MUSCULOSKELETAL SYSTEM

As you are undoubtedly aware, sedentary aging is unkind to our musculoskeletal system. Unless we perform regular strength exercise, we lose muscle and bone, beginning as early as our twenties and progressing throughout our lives.

Muscle loss, referred to as sarcopenia, is largely the result of reduced muscle-building proteins, and bone loss, called osteoporosis, is associated with reduced bone-building proteins.

You could therefore conclude that it is important to eat sufficient protein to maintain the essential cellular components of your muscles and bones. Although adequate protein intake without appropriate strength exercise is ineffective for maintaining your muscle and bone tissue, the opposite is also true. That is, your strength-training program will not be as productive if you take in too little dietary protein.

Unfortunately, there is another factor associated with the aging process that reduces protein availability to our muscle cells. For reasons that are not fully understood, as we advance in age, our muscle tissue absorbs less of the protein that we eat. Recent research has shown that a 70-year-old individual may be less than 50 percent as efficient at assimilating amino acids (muscle building blocks) from the protein he or she eats as a 30-year-old individual. In other words, even if a middle-aged man or woman is eating the recommended amount of dietary protein, approximately half of the amino acid building blocks are unavailable to the muscle cells that need them.

It would therefore appear that as we progress through the aging process, we should eat more protein-rich foods. For example, the recommended protein intake for an adult woman is approximately 50 grams per day. Let's assume that a 30-year-old woman ingests this amount on a daily basis and that she can utilize all 50 grams of the tissue-building protein. However, a 70-year-old woman is likely to assimilate only 50 percent of her daily protein intake. She may also eat 50 grams of protein daily, but as far as her muscles are concerned, she is only providing 25 grams of protein, which is inadequate for tissue maintenance. In order to supply her muscle cells with sufficient protein, she would need to eat about 100 grams of protein per day (100 grams of protein × 50% utilization = 50 grams of protein).

Because people of different body sizes need different amounts of protein, the daily protein guidelines are typically presented in grams of protein per pound of body weight. A general recommendation is about 0.4 gram of protein for each pound of body weight. Using this equation, a woman who weighs 125 pounds should eat about 50 grams of protein per day (125 pounds × 0.4 gram of protein per pound = 50 grams of protein). However, due to less-efficient amino acid synthesis as we age, we suggest the following adjusted guidelines for minimum daily protein intake.

RECOMMENDED PROTEIN INTAKE FOR A 125-POUND WOMAN

AGE	GRAMS PER POUND OF BODY WEIGHT	GRAMS PER DAY
30 years	0.40 to 0.45	50 to 56
40 years	0.45 to 0.50	56 to 62
50 years	0.50 to 0.55	62 to 68
60 years	0.55 to 0.60	68 to 74
70 years	0.60 to 0.65	74 to 80

What food sources are best for attaining more muscle- and bone-building protein? Fish, turkey, and chicken lead the list for those who eat meat. As you will see in the table "Standard and Supplemental Sources of Protein," just 6 ounces of most fish, white turkey, and white chicken provide about 45 grams of protein. If you consume milk and dairy products, standard servings of these foods supply large amounts of protein and calcium, both of which are essential components of muscles and bones. As shown in the table, two glasses of fat-free milk supply almost 20 grams of protein, and 1 cup of low-fat cottage cheese provides approximately 20 grams of protein. Other excellent sources of dietary protein include peanuts, tree nuts, soy products, egg whites, most beans, and some grains, such as wheat germ. Additionally, there are many reasonably priced and great-tasting protein powders that can be blended with milk, juice, or water as supplemental protein sources. For example, 6 tablespoons of most commercial protein powders mixed into a glass of fat-free milk supplies almost 35 grams of protein, including all of the essential amino acids.

Recent research has also revealed that *when* you consume protein-rich foods has implications for how the amino acid building blocks are assimilated into your

STANDARD AND SUPPLEMENTAL SOURCES OF PROTEIN

PROTEIN SOURCE	AMOUNT	GRAMS OF PROTEIN	COMMENT
Tuna fish	6 oz	45	Easy snack
Turkey breast	6 oz	45	Low-fat meat
Chicken breast	6 oz	45	Low-fat meat
Protein powder in milk	6 Tbsp in 1 cup	35	Easy to blend
Low-fat cottage cheese	1 cup	20	High in calcium
Peanut butter	4 Tbsp	15	High in good oils
Tree nuts	½ cup	15	High in good oils
Yogurt smoothie	1 cup	10	High in calcium
Egg whites	2 eggs	10	No fat
Fat-free milk	1 cup	10	High in calcium
Wheat germ	5 Tbsp	10	High in good oils
Soy milk	8 oz	8	Vegan alternative
Tofu	8 oz	8	Vegan alternative

muscles. Even if you attain plenty of protein from your major meals, the muscle-building process is enhanced when you ingest moderate amounts of protein, such as a glass of milk or a container of yogurt, within 1 hour after completing your strength-training session. We therefore suggest that you plan to consume a protein-rich snack shortly after you perform your strength exercises.

In fact, it is advisable to spread your protein intake somewhat evenly throughout the day, rather than eating large amounts of protein at one particular meal, such as dinner. Eating too much protein at one time can actually place additional stress on your kidneys, so try to distribute your protein intake throughout the day. For example, you might arrange your protein consumption in accordance with the recommendations presented in the table below. Each meal and snack contains moderate amounts of pro-

SAMPLE DAILY PROTEIN CONSUMPTION BASED ON THREE MEALS AND THREE SNACKS

MEAL/SNACK	PROTEIN SOURCE	APPROXIMATE GRAMS OF PROTEIN
Breakfast	1 bowl oatmeal/banana 1 cup fat-free milk	10
Midmorning snack	1 cup yogurt	10
Lunch	Peanut butter and jelly sandwich 1 cup apple juice	15
Midafternoon snack	½ cup cottage cheese/fruit	10
Dinner	Tossed salad 6 ounces baked chicken 1 cup baked beans 1 baked potato 2 cups grape juice 1 cup apple crisp	45
Midevening snack	1 cup orange juice with 2 tablespoons protein powder	10

tein that accumulate over the course of a day. The fairly evenly distributed protein sources presented in this table supply approximately 100 total grams of daily protein. Of course, this is simply a sample menu that you should adjust according to your personal protein requirements and dietary preferences.

One thing that we have consistently observed among our fitness program participants is that when they focus more on eating healthy foods, they have less interest in eating unhealthy foods. That is, when they eat more of the foods associated with muscle development, they eat less of the foods associated with fat deposition. We have also observed that people who perform regular strength exercise pay more attention to proper nutrition. Once you personally experience the physical effects of sensible strength training, we believe that you will find yourself making healthier food selections, thereby enjoying a double benefit from your exercise program.

WHEN AND HOW MUCH?

Based on our research with the *Hunger/Fullness Program* developed by Suzie Townsend, MS, RD, in Dallas, we propose a simple suggestion for when to eat and when not to eat. Basically, eat when you are hungry, and don't eat when you are full. Try using our five-point scale.

- Level One: Very hungry
- Level Two: A little hungry
- Level Three: Not hungry/not full, just right
- Level Four: A little full
- Level Five: Very full

Your main objective is to stay around Level Three, feeling just right. When you begin to feel a little hungry (Level Two), eat healthy/nutritious foods until you feel a little full (Level Four). Try to avoid feeling very hungry (Level One) because the typical response is to eat too much and then feel very full (Level Five), which obviously should be avoided on any fat-loss program. Although it may sound somewhat elementary, we have had excellent results with this simple and sensible approach to calorie control. When you feel a little full, stop eating—you will then feel even better. If all else fails, give it a try, and we think you will be pleasantly rewarded.

LOOKING BACK . . . HINDSIGHT IS 20/20

Diet plans are seldom synonymous with healthy eating patterns. Most diets require a significant reduction in calories resulting in both fat loss and muscle loss. They often provide too few nutrients for optimum physical function and almost always lead to a lower resting metabolic rate. For these and many other reasons, reduced-calorie diet plans have a very low (5 percent) success rate with respect to permanent weight loss.

We support the MyPyramid eating plan nutritional recommendations developed by the U.S. Department of Agriculture, as well as the sample meals (starting on page 164) designed by registered dietitians to accommodate the USDA guidelines at three different daily calorie levels (2,800, 2,200, or 1,600 calories/day). Depending on your size and caloric requirements, these well-balanced meal plans should provide all of the essential nutrients necessary for your muscle-building workouts, while concurrently enhancing your rate of fat loss. Just remember that your main emphasis is the exercise component of the Get Stronger, Feel Younger Plan, and that the sample menus are simply meant to complement your muscle-building activity.

We definitely recommend drinking plenty of water (eight glasses or more daily), and we encourage you to eat more protein-rich foods, especially if you are past your thirties. Try to distribute your protein sources throughout the day, and be sure to consume a protein snack within an hour after completing your strength-training session.

Finally, make an effort to eat when you *begin* to feel hungry and to stop eating when you *begin* to feel full. Don't let yourself become *very* hungry, and try to keep yourself from becoming *very* full. You should find that a regular strength-training program will help you better regulate your eating behavior.

MENU 1

	FOOD	GROUP ONE (1,600 CALORIES PER DAY) PORTION/ CALORIES	GROUP TWO (2,200 CALORIES PER DAY) PORTION/ CALORIES	GROUP THREE (2,800 CALORIES PER DAY) PORTION/ CALORIES
BREAKFAST	Waffles	2 waffles/174	2 waffles/174	2 waffles/174
	Butter	1 Tbsp/102	1 Tbsp/102	1 Tbsp/102
	Peanut butter	2 Tbsp/188	2 Tbsp/188	2 Tbsp/188
	Banana	1 small/93	1 small/93	1 small/93
	Fat-free milk	8 oz/86	8 oz/86	8 oz/86
	Peach	—	—	1 fruit/42
SNACK	Fat-free wheat crackers	—	16 crackers/160	16 crackers/160
LUNCH	Tuna fish	2 oz/73	3 oz/110	3 oz/110
	Mayo	1 Tbsp/100	1 Tbsp/100	1 Tbsp/100
	Wheat bread	2 slices/130	2 slices/130	2 slices/130
	Lettuce and tomato	—	½ cup/10	½ cup/10
	Fat-free milk	8 oz/86	8 oz/86	8 oz/86
	Apple	—	1 fruit/80	1 fruit/80
SNACK	Pear	1 fruit/100	1 fruit/100	1 fruit/100
DINNER	Fat-free milk	8 oz/86	8 oz/86	8 oz/86
	Pasta	1 cup/197	1 cup/197	1½ cups/296
	Tomato sauce	½ cup/71	½ cup/71	1 cup/142
	Zucchini	½ cup/14	½ cup/14	½ cup/14
	Ground turkey	2 oz/84	2 oz/84	3 oz/126
	Garlic bread	—	1 slice/82	2 slices/161
	with butter	—	1 Tbsp/102	1 Tbsp/102
SNACK	Celery sticks	½ cup/10	½ cup/10	½ cup/10

MENU 2

	FOOD	GROUP ONE (1,600 CALORIES PER DAY) PORTION/CALORIES	GROUP TWO (2,200 CALORIES PER DAY) PORTION/CALORIES	GROUP THREE (2,800 CALORIES PER DAY) PORTION/CALORIES
BREAKFAST	Fat-free vanilla yogurt	8 oz/206	8 oz/206	8 oz/206
	Peach	1 fruit/40	1 fruit/40	1 fruit/40
	Granola cereal	1 oz/129	2 oz/257	3 oz/386
	Orange juice	—	—	6 oz/86
LUNCH	Wheat bread	2 slices/130	2 slices/130	2 slices/130
	Chicken	2 oz/112	3 oz/168	3 oz/168
	Fat-free milk	8 oz/86	8 oz/86	8 oz/86
	Mixed vegetables	½ cup/54	1 cup/107	1½ cups/161
	Mayo	—	—	1 Tbsp/100
SNACK	English muffin	1 muffin/133	1 muffin/133	1 muffin/133
	Butter	1 Tbsp/102	1 Tbsp/102	1 Tbsp/102
DINNER	Fat-free milk	8 oz/86	8 oz/86	8 oz/86
	Roast turkey	3 oz/161	3 oz/161	4 oz/215
	Bread stuffing	½ cup/178	1 cup/356	1 cup/356
	Green beans	½ cup/19	½ cup/19	½ cup/19
	Corn	½ cup/66	½ cup/66	½ cup/66
SNACK	Fruit cocktail	½ cup/54	1 cup/108	1 cup/108
	Fat-free crackers	—	8 crackers/80	16 crackers/160

MENU 3

	FOOD	GROUP ONE (1,600 CALORIES PER DAY) PORTION/ CALORIES	GROUP TWO (2,200 CALORIES PER DAY) PORTION/ CALORIES	GROUP THREE (2,800 CALORIES PER DAY) PORTION/ CALORIES
BREAKFAST	English muffin	1 muffin/133	1 muffin/133	1 muffin/133
	Fat-free vanilla yogurt	1 cup/206	1 cup/206	1 cup/206
	Orange juice	6 oz/86	12 oz/172	12 oz/172
	Low-fat granola	—	2 oz/220	3 oz/330
LUNCH	Hummus	½ cup/208	½ cup/208	1 cup/416
	Pita bread (6")	1 piece/165	1 piece/165	1 piece/165
	Fat-free frozen yogurt	1 cup/191	1 cup/191	1 cup/191
	Strawberries	½ cup/25	½ cup/25	1 cup/50
	Angel food cake	—	—	⅙ of cake/146
SNACK	Chips Ahoy! cookies	4 cookies/123	4 cookies/123	4 cookies/123
DINNER	Fat-free milk	1 cup/86	1 cup/86	1 cup/86
	Baked chicken	4 oz/223	5 oz/279	5 oz/279
	Corn	½ cup/66	1 cup/132	1 cup/132
	Peas	—	—	½ cup/62
	Oven-fried sweet potatoes	1 cup/176	1 cup/176	1 cup/176

MENU 4

	FOOD	GROUP ONE (1,600 CALORIES PER DAY) PORTION/ CALORIES	GROUP TWO (2,200 CALORIES PER DAY) PORTION/ CALORIES	GROUP THREE (2,800 CALORIES PER DAY) PORTION/ CALORIES
BREAKFAST	Grapefruit	½ fruit/60	½ fruit/60	½ fruit/60
	Bagel	1 small/195	1 large/303	1 large/303
	Butter	—	1 Tbsp/102	1 Tbsp/102
	Fat-free vanilla yogurt	8 oz/206	8 oz/206	8 oz/206
LUNCH	Chicken salad			
	Chicken breast	2 oz/112	3 oz/168	4 oz/224
	Celery	½ cup/10	½ cup/10	½ cup/10
	Mayo	1 Tbsp/100	1 Tbsp/100	1 Tbsp/100
	Hearty roll	1 roll/152	1 roll/152	1 roll/152
	Fat-free milk	1 cup/86	1 cup/86	1 cup/86
	Side salad	—	—	1 cup/22
	Ranch dressing	—	—	1 Tbsp/60
SNACK	Banana	1 small/93	1 large/125	1 large/125
DINNER	Fat-free milk	1 cup/86	1 cup/86	1 cup/86
	Pork stir-fry			
	Pork	3 oz/206	3 oz/206	3 oz/206
	Red and green peppers	½ cup/20	1 cup/40	1 cup/40
	Broccoli	½ cup/10	½ cup/10	½ cup/10
	Peanut oil	1 Tbsp/119	1 Tbsp/119	1 Tbsp/119
	Brown rice	1 cup/218	1 cup/218	1½ cups/327
SNACK	Graham crackers	—	5 crackers/75	10 crackers/150
	Apple juice	—	—	6 oz/87

MENU 5

	FOOD	GROUP ONE (1,600 CALORIES PER DAY) PORTION/ CALORIES	GROUP TWO (2,200 CALORIES PER DAY) PORTION/ CALORIES	GROUP THREE (2,800 CALORIES PER DAY) PORTION/ CALORIES
BREAKFAST	Orange juice	6 oz/86	6 oz/86	12 oz/172
	Honey Bunches of Oats cereal	2 oz/223	2 oz/223	3 oz/335
	Fat-free milk	1 cup/86	1 cup/86	1 cup/86
LUNCH	Turkey	2 oz/107	3 oz/161	3 oz/161
	Swiss cheese	1 oz/95	1 oz/95	1 oz/95
	Tomato	¼ cup/9	¼ cup/9	¼ cup/9
	Roll	1 roll/152	1 roll/152	1 roll/152
	Mayo	—	1 Tbsp/100	1 Tbsp/100
	Grapes	½ cup/30	½ cup/30	½ cup/30
	Vegetable juice	6 oz/34	12 oz/68	12 oz/68
	Carrot sticks	½ cup/28	½ cup/28	1 cup/56
	Ranch dressing	1 Tbsp/60	1 Tbsp/60	1 Tbsp/60
SNACK	Fat-free vanilla yogurt	8 oz/206	8 oz/206	8 oz/206
	Low-fat granola	—	2 oz/220	3 oz/330
DINNER	Chicken breast	3 oz/168	3 oz/168	4 oz/224
	Salsa	¼ cup/18	¼ cup/18	¼ cup/18
	Cheddar cheese	1 oz/114	1 oz/114	1 oz/114
	Spanish rice	1 cup/216	1½ cups/324	1½ cups/324
SNACK	Apple	—	1 fruit/80	1 fruit/80

MENU 6

	FOOD	GROUP ONE (1,600 CALORIES PER DAY) PORTION/ CALORIES	GROUP TWO (2,200 CALORIES PER DAY) PORTION/ CALORIES	GROUP THREE (2,800 CALORIES PER DAY) PORTION/ CALORIES
BREAKFAST	English muffin	1 muffin/133	1 muffin/133	1 muffin/133
	Butter	—	1 Tbsp/102	1 Tbsp/102
	Fat-free vanilla yogurt	8 oz/206	8 oz/206	8 oz/206
	Raisins	¼ cup/107	¼ cup/107	¼ cup/107
	Low-fat granola	2 oz/220	3 oz/330	4 oz/440
LUNCH	Grilled cheese			
	Wheat bread	2 slices/130	2 slices/130	2 slices/130
	American cheese	2 oz/186	2 oz/186	2 oz/186
	Tomatoes	½ cup/19	½ cup/19	½ cup/19
	Butter	1 Tbsp/102	1 Tbsp/102	1 Tbsp/102
	Mixed green salad	—	1 cup/9	2 cups/18
	Chickpeas	—	—	1 cup/286
	Cranberry juice	6 oz/97	12 oz/194	12 oz/194
SNACK	Graham crackers	—	12 crackers/180	18 crackers/270
	Peanut butter	—	1 Tbsp/94	1 Tbsp/94
DINNER	Haddock	5 oz/169	5 oz/169	6 oz/203
	Baked potato	1 potato/133	1 potato/133	1 potato/133
	—stuffed with broccoli	½ cup/26	½ cup/26	½ cup/26
	Fat-free shredded cheese	2 oz/81	2 oz/81	2 oz/81
	Honeydew melon	—	—	½ cup/30

MENU 7

	FOOD	GROUP ONE (1,600 CALORIES PER DAY) PORTION/CALORIES	GROUP TWO (2,200 CALORIES PER DAY) PORTION/CALORIES	GROUP THREE (2,800 CALORIES PER DAY) PORTION/CALORIES
BREAKFAST	Bagel	1 small/195	1 large/303	1 large/303
	Butter	—	1 Tbsp/102	1 Tbsp/102
	Cranberry juice	6 oz/97	12 oz/194	12 oz/194
	Banana	—	—	1 small/92
LUNCH	Tuna	2 oz/73	2 oz/73	3 oz/110
	Mayo	1 Tbsp/100	1 Tbsp/100	1 Tbsp/100
	Wheat bread	2 slices/130	2 slices/130	2 slices/130
	Lettuce	½ cup/3	½ cup/3	1 cup/6
	Tomatoes	¼ cup/10	¼ cup/10	½ cup/20
	Apple	1 fruit/80	1 fruit/80	1 fruit/80
	Fat-free milk	8 oz/86	8 oz/86	8 oz/86
	Graham cracker	—	—	12 crackers/180
DINNER	Ham, low-sodium	3 oz/155	4 oz/206	4 oz/206
	Squash	½ cup/18	1 cup/36	1 cup/36
	Baked potato	1 potato/133	1 potato/133	1 potato/133
	Butter	1 Tbsp/102	1 Tbsp/102	1 Tbsp/102
	Fat-free milk	8 oz/86	8 oz/86	8 oz/86
SNACK	Fat-free vanilla yogurt	8 oz/206	8 oz/206	8 oz/206
	Grape-Nuts cereal	2 oz/204	3 oz/306	3 oz/306

MENU 8

	FOOD	GROUP ONE (1,600 CALORIES PER DAY) PORTION/ CALORIES	GROUP TWO (2,200 CALORIES PER DAY) PORTION/ CALORIES	GROUP THREE (2,800 CALORIES PER DAY) PORTION/ CALORIES
BREAKFAST	Cheerios	2 oz/207	2 oz/207	2 oz/207
	Fat-free milk	8 oz/86	8 oz/86	8 oz/86
	Apple juice	6 oz/87	6 oz/87	12 oz/174
	Bagel	½ small/98	1 small/195	1 large/303
	Cream cheese	1 oz/99	1 oz/99	2 oz/198
	Sugar	—	—	1 Tbsp/46
SNACK	Orange	1 fruit/70	1 fruit/70	1 fruit/70
LUNCH	Wheat bread	2 slices/130	2 slices/130	2 slices/130
	Turkey breast	2 oz/107	3 oz/161	3 oz/161
	Mayo	1 Tbsp/100	1 Tbsp/100	1 Tbsp/100
	Fat-free milk	8 oz/86	8 oz/86	8 oz/86
	Side salad	—	1 cup/22	1 cup/22
	Ranch salad dressing	—	1 Tbsp/60	2 Tbsp/120
	Apple	—	1 fruit/80	1 fruit/80
SNACK	Celery and carrot sticks	½ cup/18	1 cup/36	1 cup/36
	Graham crackers	—	4 crackers/60	4 crackers/60
DINNER	Fat-free milk	8 oz/86	8 oz/86	8 oz/86
	Chicken breast	3 oz/168	3 oz/168	4 oz/224
	Dinner roll	1 roll/107	1 roll/107	1 roll/107
	Brown rice	—	½ cup/109	½ cup/109
	Green beans	½ cup/20	—	½ cup/20
	Corn	½ cup/66	½ cup/66	½ cup/66
	Butter	—	1 Tbsp/102	2 Tbsp/204

MENU 9

	FOOD	GROUP ONE (1,600 CALORIES PER DAY) PORTION/ CALORIES	GROUP TWO (2,200 CALORIES PER DAY) PORTION/ CALORIES	GROUP THREE (2,800 CALORIES PER DAY) PORTION/ CALORIES
BREAKFAST	Special K cereal	2 oz/210	2 oz/210	4 oz/420
	Fat-free milk	1 cup/86	1 cup/86	1 cup/86
	Apple juice	12 oz/175	12 oz/175	12 oz/175
LUNCH	Wheat bread	2 slices/130	2 slices/130	2 slices/130
	Ham	2 oz/103	3 oz/155	3 oz/155
	American cheese	2 oz/186	2 oz/186	2 oz/186
	Lettuce	—	½ cup/3	1 cup/6
	Tomato	—	¼ cup/10	½ cup/19
	Banana	—	1 small/93	1 large/125
SNACK	Fat-free crackers	8 crackers/80	16 crackers/160	16 crackers/160
DINNER	Fat-free milk	1 cup/86	1 cup/86	1 cup/86
	Haddock	3 oz/101	3 oz/101	4 oz/135
	Butter	—	1 Tbsp/102	1 Tbsp/102
	Bread crumbs	—	½ cup/220	½ cup/220
	Baked potato	1 potato/133	1 potato/133	1 potato/133
	Mixed vegetables	1 cup/107	1 cup/107	1 cup/107
SNACK	Bagel	½ small/98	1 small/195	1 small/195
	Butter	1 Tbsp/102	—	1 Tbsp/102

MENU 10

	FOOD	GROUP ONE (1,600 CALORIES PER DAY) PORTION/CALORIES	GROUP TWO (2,200 CALORIES PER DAY) PORTION/CALORIES	GROUP THREE (2,800 CALORIES PER DAY) PORTION/CALORIES
BREAKFAST	Scrambled eggs			
	Whole egg	1 egg/75	2 eggs/150	2 eggs/150
	American cheese	1 oz/93	1 oz/93	1 oz/93
	Fat-free milk	4 oz/43	4 oz/43	4 oz/43
	Orange juice	6 oz/86	12 oz/172	12 oz/172
	English muffin	1 muffin/133	1 muffin/133	2 muffins/266
	Butter	—	1 Tbsp/102	1 Tbsp/102
LUNCH	Tuna fish	3 oz/109	3 oz/109	4 oz/145
	Wheat bread	2 slices/130	2 slices/130	2 slices/130
	Mayo	1 Tbsp/100	1 Tbsp/100	1 Tbsp/100
	Celery sticks	½ cup/10	1 cup/20	1 cup/20
	Peanut butter	2 Tbsp/188	2 Tbsp/188	2 Tbsp/188
	Fat-free milk	1 cup/86	1 cup/86	1 cup/86
SNACK	Peach	1 fruit/40	1 fruit/40	1 fruit/40
DINNER	Pasta salad			
	Pasta	1 cup/197	2 cups/394	2 cups/394
	Red and green pepper	½ cup/12	½ cup/12	1 cup/24
	Celery and cucumber	½ cup/8	½ cup/8	½ cup/8
	Fat-free Italian dressing	1 Tbsp/10	1 Tbsp/10	1 Tbsp/10
SNACK	Fat-free vanilla yogurt	8 oz/206	8 oz/206	8 oz/206
	Low-fat granola	—	1 oz/128	1 oz/128
	Raisins	—	—	¼ cup/107

MENU 11

	FOOD	GROUP ONE (1,600 CALORIES PER DAY) PORTION/ CALORIES	GROUP TWO (2,200 CALORIES PER DAY) PORTION/ CALORIES	GROUP THREE (2,800 CALORIES PER DAY) PORTION/ CALORIES
BREAKFAST	Grape-Nuts cereal	1 oz/102	2 oz/204	2 oz/204
	OR Cheerios	2 oz/207	2 oz/207	3 oz/311
	Fat-free milk	1 cup/86	1 cup/86	1 cup/86
	Wheat toast	—	—	1 slice/65
	Orange	1 fruit/70	1 fruit/70	1 fruit/70
	Butter	—	—	1 Tbsp/102
LUNCH	Wheat bread	2 slices/130	2 slices/130	2 slices/130
	Tuna	2 oz/73	2 oz/73	3 oz/110
	Mayo	—	1 Tbsp/100	1 Tbsp/100
	Celery, chopped	¼ cup/5	¼ cup/5	¼ cup/5
	Carrots, chopped	—	—	¼ cup/14
	Lettuce	½ cup/3	½ cup/3	½ cup/3
	Tomato	—	—	½ cup/19
	Apple juice	6 oz/87	6 oz/87	12 oz/174
SNACK	Fat-free crackers	—	12 crackers/120	12 crackers/120
	Peanut butter	—	2 Tbsp/188	2 Tbsp/188
DINNER	Salmon, grilled	3 oz/118	3 oz/118	3 oz/118
	Tossed salad	1 cup/22	1 cup/22	1 cup/22
	Olive oil	1 Tbsp/119	1 Tbsp/119	1 Tbsp/119
	Broccoli	½ cup/26	1 cup/52	1 cup/52
	Dinner roll	1 roll/107	1 roll/107	1 roll/107
	Vanilla ice cream	½ cup/133	½ cup/133	½ cup/133
SNACK	Fat-free vanilla yogurt	8 oz/206	8 oz/206	8 oz/206
	Apple	—	1 fruit/80	1 fruit/80

MENU 12

FOOD		GROUP ONE (1,600 CALORIES PER DAY) PORTION/ CALORIES	GROUP TWO (2,200 CALORIES PER DAY) PORTION/ CALORIES	GROUP THREE (2,800 CALORIES PER DAY) PORTION/ CALORIES
BREAKFAST	Hard-cooked egg	1 egg/75	1 egg/75	1 egg/75
	Wheat toast	2 slices/130	2 slices/130	2 slices/130
	Butter	1 Tbsp/102	1 Tbsp/102	1 Tbsp/102
	Grapefruit juice	6 oz/70	12 oz/140	12 oz/140
	Fat-free vanilla yogurt	8 oz/206	8 oz/206	8 oz/206
LUNCH	Three-bean salad	1 cup/160	1 cup/160	1½ cups/204
	Fat-free milk	1 cup/86	1 cup/86	1 cup/86
	Pita bread (6")	1 piece/165	1 piece/165	1 piece/165
	Side salad	1 cup/22	2 cups/44	2 cups/44
	Ranch salad dressing	1 Tbsp/60	1 Tbsp/60	1 Tbsp/60
	Cantaloupe	½ cup/29	½ cup/29	1 cup/57
SNACK	Bagel	—	—	½ small/98
	Cream cheese	—	—	1 oz/99
DINNER	Stir-fry			
	Rice	1 cup/218	1½ cups/327	2 cups/436
	Chicken breast	2 oz/112	3 oz/168	3 oz/168
	Red and green pepper and onion	1 cup/24	1 cup/24	1½ cups/36
	Fat-free milk	8 oz/86	8 oz/86	8 oz/86
SNACK	Vanilla wafers	10 wafers/190	10 wafers/190	10 wafers/190

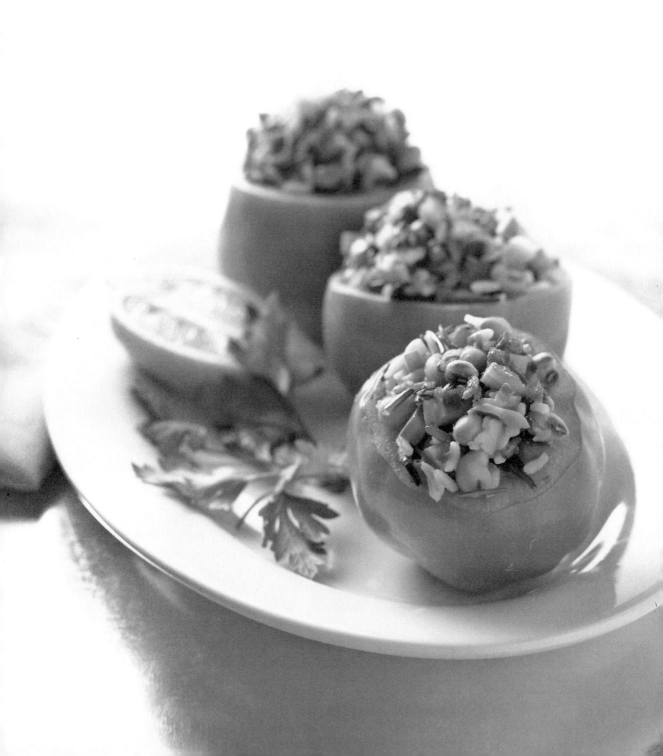

CHAPTER 11

RECIPES

Nutritionists tell us that most people eat essentially the same six to 10 basic meal plans most days of the year. Assuming these dinners are well-balanced nutritionally, there is no problem from a health perspective, but eating the same meals repeatedly can become boring. For a more varied and exciting mealtime, try the more than 30 delicious recipes included in this chapter, from soups and salads to entrées and desserts.

In addition to easy-to-find ingredients and easy-to-implement mixing/cooking instructions, each recipe contains pertinent per-serving nutritional information, such as the number of calories and the amount of protein, carbohydrate, fat, cholesterol, sodium, and fiber.

If you are in the market for new and nutritious menu items, you will be pleasantly surprised by these innovative and delicious recipes for healthy eating. Try one or two new recipes a week, and see how many you add to your previous list of favorite meals and snacks.

Smoothies

YOGURT-BERRY SMOOTHIE

1 cup frozen berries, such as blueberries, raspberries, or strawberries

½ cup low-fat yogurt (any flavor)

½ cup orange juice or other juice

Place the berries, yogurt, and orange juice in a blender and pulse for 30 seconds. Blend for 30 seconds, or until smooth.

Makes 1 serving

PER SERVING: *185 calories, 8 g protein, 35 g carbohydrates, 2 g fat, 7 mg cholesterol, 90 mg sodium, 3 g dietary fiber*

BANANA SMOOTHIE

2 bananas

2 cups 1% milk

1–2 tablespoons chocolate or other flavor syrup

½ cup ice cubes

In a food processor or blender, combine the bananas, milk, syrup, and ice cubes. Process until frothy.

Makes 4 servings

PER SERVING: *119 calories, 5 g protein, 23 g carbohydrate, 1 g fat, 5 mg cholesterol, 65 mg sodium, 2 g dietary fiber*

Soups

CALIFORNIA CHICKEN SOUP

3 cans (14¾ ounces each) fat-free chicken broth

2 cups water

1 pound cooked cubed chicken breast

2 medium carrots, chopped

1 small onion, chopped

1¾ teaspoons ground lemon pepper

1 teaspoon dried oregano

1 package (9 ounces) cheese tortellini

2 stalks broccoli, cut into florets (2 cups)

Freshly grated Parmesan cheese (optional)

In a large pot over medium-high heat, combine the broth, water, chicken, carrots, onion, lemon pepper, and oregano and bring to a boil. Add the tortellini. Reduce the heat to low and simmer for 25 minutes. Add the broccoli and cook for 5 minutes, or until the broccoli and tortellini are tender. Sprinkle with the cheese, if using.

Makes 6 servings

PER SERVING: *287 calories, 33 g protein, 17 g carbohydrates, 9 g fat, 75 mg cholesterol, 460 mg sodium, 2 g dietary fiber*

SOUTHWEST CHOWDER

4 ears corn, husks and silks removed

2 dried chipotle chile peppers (wear plastic gloves when handling)

2 teaspoons olive oil

3 ribs celery, chopped

1 onion, chopped

2 cloves garlic, minced

1½ teaspoons ground cumin

5 cups fat-free chicken broth

8 ounces Yukon gold potatoes, cubed

2 bay leaves

1 butternut squash, peeled and cubed

1 roasted red pepper, chopped

¼ cup unbleached all-purpose flour

2 cups 1% milk

8 oyster crackers (optional)

Cook the corn in a large pot of boiling water for 3 minutes, or until tender. Drain and set aside until cool enough to handle. Slice 2 cups kernels off the cobs and set aside; reserve the cobs.

Place the chile peppers in a small bowl. Cover with hot water and let stand for 10 minutes, or until soft. Remove and discard the stems and seeds. Finely chop the peppers; reserve the soaking liquid.

Warm the oil in a large saucepan over medium heat. Add the celery, onion, garlic, and cumin and cook, stirring frequently, for 6 minutes, or until the vegetables are soft and tender. Stir in the broth, potatoes, bay leaves, reserved corn cobs, chipotle soaking liquid, and finely chopped chipotle peppers. Cook for 10 minutes. Add the squash and corn. Cook, stirring occasionally, for 15 minutes, or until the vegetables are tender. Remove and discard the bay leaves and the corn cobs. Stir in the roasted pepper.

Place the flour in a medium bowl. Slowly whisk in the milk until smooth. Stir into the soup and cook, stirring frequently, for 7 minutes, or until slightly thickened. Serve with the oyster crackers, if using.

Makes 8 servings

PER SERVING: *173 calories, 10 g protein, 30 g carbohydrates, 3 g fat, 5 mg cholesterol, 160 mg sodium, 4 g dietary fiber*

EASY MINESTRONE

- 1 tablespoon olive oil
- 3 ribs celery, chopped
- 1 onion, chopped
- 3 cups water
- 3 packets or cubes (3 teaspoons) beef bouillon
- 1 can (28 ounces) whole tomatoes, chopped
- 2 teaspoons dried basil
- 2 teaspoons chopped parsley
- 1 teaspoon dried oregano
- ½ teaspoon ground black pepper
- 1 bay leaf
- 2 medium potatoes, chopped
- 2 medium carrots, chopped
- 2 cans (14–19 ounces each) kidney beans, rinsed and drained
- ½ cup small shell pasta
- Parmesan cheese and/or sour cream

Heat the oil in a medium saucepan over medium heat. Add the celery and onion and cook for 10 minutes, or until soft but not brown. Add the water, bouillon, tomatoes (with juice), basil, parsley, oregano, pepper, and bay leaf. Bring to a boil. Reduce the heat to low, cover, and simmer for 25 minutes.

Add the potatoes and carrots, cover, and simmer for 15 minutes, or until the vegetables are tender. Add the beans and pasta and cook for 12 minutes, or until the pasta is al dente. Remove and discard the bay leaf. Serve with a sprinkling of cheese or a swirl of sour cream.

Makes 12 servings

PER SERVING: *120 calories, 6 g protein, 23 g carbohydrates, 2 g fat, 0 mg cholesterol, 440 mg sodium, 5 g dietary fiber*

CHICKEN PARMESAN

¼ cup liquid egg substitute

1 cup Italian or whole wheat bread crumbs

½ cup (2 ounces) grated Parmesan cheese

2 tablespoons chopped parsley

2–3 cloves garlic, minced

4 boneless skinless chicken breast halves, pounded to ½" thickness

1 cup tomato sauce

1 cup (4 ounces) shredded reduced-fat mozzarella cheese

Preheat the oven to 375°F. Coat a baking sheet with cooking spray.

Place the egg substitute in a shallow dish. In another shallow dish, combine the bread crumbs, Parmesan, parsley, and garlic. Dip the chicken in the egg substitute, then dredge in the bread-crumb mixture. Place the chicken on the prepared baking sheet.

Bake for 10 minutes. Place ¼ cup of the tomato sauce over each chicken breast half and top each with ¼ cup of the mozzarella. Bake for 20 minutes, or until a thermometer inserted in the thickest portion registers 160°F and the juices run clear and the cheese is melted.

Makes 4 servings

PER SERVING: *328 calories, 53 g protein, 7 g carbohydrates, 10 g fat, 120 mg cholesterol, 861 mg sodium, 1 g dietary fiber*

THAI CHICKEN STIR-SIZZLE

Peanut Sauce

- ¾ cup water
- ¼ cup + 2 tablespoons creamy peanut butter
- 3 tablespoons soy sauce
- 2 tablespoons rice vinegar
- ¾ teaspoon red-pepper flakes

Stir-Sizzle

- 6 ounces soba noodles or linguine
- 1 teaspoon toasted sesame oil

- 1 pound boneless, skinless chicken breast, sliced crosswise into ½" pieces
- 1 bunch scallions, sliced diagonally into 1" pieces
- 3 cloves garlic, minced
- 2 teaspoons grated fresh ginger
- 1 cup snow peas
- 1 red bell pepper, cut into thin strips
- 1 medium carrot, shredded
- 2 tablespoons chopped fresh cilantro

To make the peanut sauce: In a blender, combine the water, peanut butter, soy sauce, and vinegar and process until smooth. Add the pepper flakes and set aside.

To make the stir-sizzle: Prepare the noodles according to package directions. Drain and return to the pot.

Meanwhile, warm the oil in a large nonstick skillet over medium-high heat. Add the chicken and cook for 4 minutes, or until no longer pink. Add the scallions, garlic, and ginger and cook for 2 minutes, stirring often and being careful not to let the garlic burn. Add the snow peas, pepper, and carrot and cook for 2 minutes. Stir in the peanut sauce and pour over the noodles in the pot. Sprinkle with the cilantro and toss to coat. Place over heat for 2 minutes, or until heated through.

Makes 6 servings

PER SERVING: *315 calories, 27 g protein, 31 g carbohydrates, 10 g fat, 45 mg cholesterol, 870 mg sodium, 3 g dietary fiber*

MEXICAN CASSEROLE

2 cups broken low-fat corn chips

1 pound ground turkey breast

1 onion, chopped

1 can (10¾ ounces) low-fat cream of chicken soup

¾ cup salsa

¾ cup (3 ounces) shredded low-fat Cheddar cheese

Preheat the oven to 350°F. Place a layer of corn chips in an 11" × 7" baking dish.

Heat a large nonstick skillet over medium-high heat. Add the turkey and onion and cook, stirring frequently, for 5 minutes, or until the turkey is no longer pink and the onion is soft. Drain if necessary. Add the soup and salsa and stir to combine.

Place a layer of turkey over the chips in the baking dish and top with a layer of cheese and a layer of chips. Repeat to use the remaining turkey, cheese, and chips, ending with cheese.

Bake for 15 minutes, or until heated through. Let stand for 5 minutes before serving.

Makes 8 servings

PER SERVING: *170 calories, 14 g protein, 9 g carbohydrates, 9 g fat, 50 mg cholesterol, 425 mg sodium, 1 g dietary fiber*

MEXICAN TURKEY MEATLOAF

1½ cups chunky medium salsa

1 egg white

1 pound ground turkey breast

1–1½ cups old-fashioned rolled oats

¼ teaspoon ground black pepper

½ cup (2 ounces) shredded reduced-fat Cheddar or soy cheese alternative

5 black olives, finely chopped

2–3 scallions, finely chopped

Preheat the oven to 350°F. Coat a loaf pan with cooking spray.

In a large bowl, combine 1 cup of the salsa and the egg white. Add the turkey and mix in by hand. Add 1 cup of the oats, mixing in by hand. Add up to ½ cup more oats if needed to reach desired consistency. Place in the prepared loaf pan (it will be a little messy), allowing ½" of space along the side of the pan. Sprinkle with the pepper. Top with the remaining ½ cup salsa.

Bake for 50 minutes. Top with the cheese, olives, and scallions. Bake for 10 minutes longer, or until a thermometer inserted in the center registers 165°F and the turkey is no longer pink.

Makes 8 servings

PER SERVING: *157 calories, 14 g protein, 10 g carbohydrate, 6 g fat, 46 mg cholesterol, 339 mg sodium, 2 g dietary fiber*

OLD-FASHIONED BEEF STEW

- 1 tablespoon olive oil
- ¼ cup unbleached all-purpose flour
- ¼ teaspoon ground black pepper
- 1½ pounds lean boneless beef round steak, trimmed of all visible fat and cut into 1" cubes
- 1 medium onion, chopped
- 2 cloves garlic, minced
- 1 teaspoon dried thyme
- 2 bay leaves
- 3 cups dry red wine or nonalcoholic red wine

- ¼ cup tomato paste
- 2 cans (14 ounces each) fat-free beef broth
- 1½ pounds baby red potatoes, quartered
- 20 baby carrots
- 16 baby pattypan squash, halved
- 1 pound shiitake mushrooms, thickly sliced
- ¼ cup chopped Italian parsley

Heat 1½ teaspoons of the oil in a Dutch oven over medium-high heat.

In a medium bowl, combine the flour and pepper. Working in batches, dredge the beef in the flour, place in the pot, and cook for 4 minutes, or until browned on all sides; do not overcrowd the pot. With a slotted spoon, remove the beef to a plate.

Add the remaining 1½ teaspoons oil to the pot. Reduce the heat to medium and add the onion, garlic, thyme, and bay leaves. Cook, stirring often, for 6 minutes, or until the onion is tender. Stir in the wine and tomato paste. With a wooden spoon, scrape up any browned bits from the bottom of the pot.

Add the broth and beef and bring to a boil. Partially cover and simmer for 1½ hours, or until the beef is tender.

Add the potatoes and carrots and simmer for 20 minutes. Add the squash, mushrooms, and parsley and simmer for 10 minutes, or until the vegetables are tender. Remove and discard the bay leaves before serving.

Makes 8 servings

PER SERVING: *330 calories, 22 g protein, 33 g carbohydrates, 6 g fat, 45 mg cholesterol, 130 mg sodium, 5 g dietary fiber*

HOME-RUN HAMBURGERS

3 tablespoons bulgur

⅓ cup boiling water

1 teaspoon olive oil

1 medium Vidalia onion, thinly sliced

1½ cups sliced shiitake mushrooms

1¼ pounds extra-lean ground beef

⅓ cup fresh bread crumbs

¼ cup chopped Italian parsley

2 tablespoons Worcestershire sauce

2 tablespoons tomato paste

2 cloves garlic, minced

1 teaspoon ground black pepper

½ teaspoon mustard powder

6 leaves red leaf lettuce

6 tomato slices

6 whole grain hamburger buns, split

Place the bulgur in a large bowl and add the water. Cover and let stand for 15 minutes, or until soft.

Heat the oil in a large nonstick skillet over medium heat. Add the onion and cook for 10 minutes, or until soft. Add the mushrooms and cook for 5 minutes, or until soft.

Drain the bulgur and return to the bowl. Stir in the beef, bread crumbs, parsley, Worcestershire sauce, tomato paste, garlic, pepper, and mustard. Shape the mixture into six 1"-thick patties.

Coat a grill rack or broiler-pan rack with cooking spray. Preheat the grill or broiler.

Cook the burgers 4" from the heat for 4 minutes per side, or until a thermometer inserted in a burger registers 160°F and the meat is no longer pink.

Place the lettuce and tomato on the bottom halves of the buns. Top with the burgers, then divide the onions and mushrooms among the burgers. Top each with the bun tops.

Makes 6 hamburgers

PER HAMBURGER: *300 calories, 27 g protein, 36 g carbohydrates, 7 g fat, 50 mg cholesterol, 350 mg sodium, 6 g dietary fiber*

PORK MEDALLIONS WITH BLACK OLIVES

1 pound pork tenderloin, trimmed, cut into 8 pieces, and pounded to ¼" thickness

½ teaspoon ground black pepper

¼–½ teaspoon salt

¼ cup unbleached or all-purpose flour

1 tablespoon olive oil

½ cup dry white wine or nonalcoholic wine

½ cup reduced-sodium chicken broth

1 tablespoon parsley

2 tablespoons sliced black olives, drained

Sprinkle the pork with the pepper and salt. Place the flour in a shallow dish. Dredge the pork in the flour, turning to coat. Shake off any excess flour.

Heat 1½ teaspoons of the oil in a large nonstick skillet over medium-high heat. Add half of the pork and cook for 2 minutes on each side, or until no longer pink. Remove to a plate and keep warm. Repeat to use the remaining oil and pork.

Return the reserved pork to the pan. Add the wine, broth, and parsley and bring to a boil. Stir in the olives and cook for 4 minutes.

Makes 4 servings

PER SERVING: *226 calories, 25 g protein, 7 g carbohydrate, 8 g fat, 74 mg cholesterol, 263 mg sodium, 0 g dietary fiber*

CAESAR KEBABS

4 small potatoes, scrubbed and halved

1 pound steak or boneless, skinless chicken breasts, cut into bite-size pieces

2 medium red and/or green bell peppers, cut into chunks

1 small onion, cut into chunks

Pinch of salt

Pinch of ground black pepper

½ cup light Caesar vinaigrette dressing

Bring a medium pot of water to a boil over high heat. Add the potatoes and cook for 20 minutes, or until fork-tender.

Coat a grill rack or broiler-pan rack with cooking spray. Preheat the grill or broiler.

In a large bowl, combine the beef and/or chicken, potatoes, bell peppers, onion, salt, and black pepper. Add the dressing and toss to coat. Alternately thread the meat and vegetables onto 4 metal skewers. Place on the prepared rack or pan and cook, turning occasionally, for 15 minutes for beef, 25 minutes for chicken, or until the meat is no longer pink.

Makes 4 servings

PER SERVING: *255 calories, 30 g protein, 30 g carbohydrate, 3 g fat, 66 mg cholesterol, 398 mg sodium, 4 g dietary fiber*

EASY PIZZA LITE

1 flour tortilla (8" diameter)

2 tablespoons pizza sauce

¼ cup (1 ounce) shredded reduced-fat mozzarella cheese

4 thin slices turkey pepperoni

Preheat the oven or toaster oven to 350°F.

Place the tortilla on a baking sheet. Spread the sauce over the tortilla. Top with the cheese and pepperoni.

Bake for 10 minutes, or until the cheese is melted.

Makes 1 serving

PER SERVING: *375 calories, 31 g protein, 31 g carbohydrate, 14 g fat, 83 mg cholesterol, 1,664 mg sodium, 0 g dietary fiber*

CRAB CAKES WITH ROASTED PEPPER SAUCE

Roasted Pepper Sauce
- 2 roasted red peppers
- ½ cup fat-free mayonnaise
- Ground black pepper

Crab Cakes
- 1 teaspoon olive oil
- ½ small onion, finely chopped
- 1 rib celery, finely chopped
- 1 egg white
- 2 tablespoons chopped Italian parsley
- 2 tablespoons fat-free mayonnaise
- 1 tablespoon lemon juice
- 1½ teaspoons crab boil seasoning
- ½ teaspoon mustard powder
- ¼ teaspoon ground paprika
- 1 pound lump crabmeat
- 1 cup fresh bread crumbs

To make the sauce: Puree the roasted peppers in a food processor or blender. Add the mayonnaise and black pepper and process briefly to combine.

To make the crab cakes: Heat the oil in a medium nonstick skillet over medium-high heat. Add the onion and celery and cook for 5 minutes, or until soft. Place in a large bowl. Stir in the egg white, parsley, mayonnaise, lemon juice, crab boil seasoning, mustard, and paprika. Stir in the crabmeat and mix thoroughly. Form into 8 patties. Roll in the bread crumbs to coat completely.

Heat a large nonstick skillet coated with cooking spray over medium-high heat. Add the crab cakes and cook for 2 minutes; cover and cook for 1 minute longer, or until browned on the bottom. Coat the tops with cooking spray and turn over. Cook for 2 minutes, uncovered, or until golden brown. Serve with the sauce.

Makes 4 servings

PER SERVING: *210 calories, 26 g protein, 19 g carbohydrates, 4 g fat, 115 mg cholesterol, 650 mg sodium, 2 g dietary fiber*

STUFFED FLOUNDER

1 tablespoon olive oil

½ pound peeled and deveined shrimp, cut up

½ teaspoon minced garlic

⅓–½ cup unseasoned dried bread crumbs

2 tablespoons grated Parmesan cheese

1 pound flounder fillets

¼ cup white wine or nonalcoholic white wine

½ tablespoon parsley

Preheat the oven to 350°F.

Heat the oil in a large skillet over medium-high heat. Add the shrimp and garlic and cook, stirring frequently, for 5 minutes, or until the shrimp is opaque. Remove to a large bowl. Add the bread crumbs and cheese and stir to combine.

Place the flounder on a work surface. Evenly divide the shrimp mixture among the fillets, spreading almost to the edge. Roll the fillets from a short end to enclose the filling. Secure with wooden picks. Place the rolls in a 13" × 9" baking dish. Pour the wine into the dish. Sprinkle with the parsley.

Bake for 15 minutes, or until the fish flakes easily.

Makes 4 servings

PER SERVING: *250 calories, 35 g protein, 7 g carbohydrate, 7 g fat, 143 mg cholesterol, 300 mg sodium, 0 g dietary fiber*

SALMON HASH

- 2 potatoes, chopped
- 1 large onion, finely chopped, with 1 tablespoon reserved for garnish
- 1 green bell pepper, finely chopped
- 1 can (15 ounces) red salmon, drained (do not use fresh)
- Creole spice, to taste
- ½ teaspoon freshly ground black pepper
- 3–4 scallions, chopped
- 1 tablespoon grated Parmesan cheese
- ¼ cup parsley, finely chopped, with 2 tablespoons reserved for garnish
- 1 teaspoon lemon peel

Place the potatoes in a microwaveable bowl. Cover with plastic wrap and microwave on high power for 3½ minutes. Let cool while preparing the other ingredients.

Heat a large nonstick skillet coated with cooking spray over medium heat. Add the onion and bell pepper and cook, stirring frequently, for 5 minutes, or until the onion is soft. Stir in the potatoes, salmon, Creole spice, and black pepper. Cook, stirring, for 5 minutes, or until the potatoes are tender and browned. Add the scallions, cheese, and parsley. Mix thoroughly. Garnish with the remaining 1 tablespoon onion, 2 tablespoons parsley, and the lemon peel.

Makes 4 servings

PER SERVING: *239 calories, 23 g protein, 23 g carbohydrate, 7 g fat, 42 mg cholesterol, 528 mg sodium, 4 g dietary fiber*

SPICY 'N' LIGHT SHRIMP CURRY

12 ounces angel hair pasta or
    1½ cups white rice

½ cup fat-free evaporated milk

½ cup fat-free sour cream

½–1 tablespoon curry powder

1 tablespoon finely chopped fresh
    basil

½ teaspoon red chili paste

2 teaspoons olive oil

1 pound medium shrimp, peeled
    and deveined

1 onion, finely chopped

1 red bell pepper, finely chopped

½ pound snow peas, trimmed

½ pound mushrooms, sliced

Prepare the pasta or rice according to package directions.

In a small bowl, combine the milk, sour cream, curry powder, basil, and chili paste. Set aside.

Heat 1 teaspoon of the oil in a large wok or nonstick skillet over medium-high heat. Add the shrimp and cook, stirring constantly, for 5 minutes, or until the shrimp are opaque. Remove to a bowl; set aside.

Heat the remaining 1 teaspoon oil in the wok. Add the onion, pepper, snow peas, and mushrooms and cook, stirring constantly, for 3 minutes, or until tender-crisp. Stir in the shrimp and reserved milk mixture and cook, stirring constantly, for 2 minutes, or until heated through. Serve in bowls over the rice or pasta.

Makes 6 servings

PER SERVING: *375 calories, 28 g protein, 56 g carbohydrate, 4 g fat, 115 mg cholesterol, 177 mg sodium, 4 g dietary fiber*

TUNA PATTIES

1 can (12 ounces) albacore tuna, drained

2 small scallions (green and white parts), finely chopped

1 egg

1 egg white

¼ teaspoon salt

2 slices low-fat Swiss or American cheese

2 whole wheat English muffins, split

2 large leaves lettuce

4 slices tomato

In a medium bowl, combine the tuna, scallions, egg, egg white, and salt. Form into 2 patties.

Heat a medium skillet coated with cooking spray over medium heat. Add the patties and cook for 2 minutes on each side, or until lightly browned.

Meanwhile, place 1 slice of cheese on 2 of the muffin halves. Toast in the toaster oven until the cheese is melted. Top the other muffin halves with tuna patties. Top with the lettuce, tomato, and the remaining muffin halves.

Makes 2 servings

PER SERVING: *442 calories, 55 g protein, 32 g carbohydrate, 10 g fat, 183 mg cholesterol, 1,033 mg sodium, 5 g dietary fiber*

Vegetarian

BLACK BEAN QUESADILLAS

1 can (14–19 ounces) no-salt black
  beans, rinsed and drained

1 teaspoon dried onion flakes

8 flour or whole wheat tortillas
  (8" in diameter)

2 cups (8 ounces) shredded low-fat
  Colby or Monterey Jack cheese

1 cup salsa (optional)

½ cup fat-free sour cream (optional)

Place the beans and onion flakes in a small saucepan over low heat and cook for 5 minutes, or until warm. Mash the beans with a spoon. Keep warm.

Meanwhile, heat a large nonstick skillet coated with cooking spray over medium heat. Place 1 tortilla in the pan and sprinkle with ¼ cup of the cheese. Cook for 2 minutes, or until the cheese melts. Spoon one-quarter of the bean mixture on top and sprinkle with ¼ cup cheese. Top with another tortilla. Carefully turn the quesadilla and cook for 2 minutes, or until browned. Repeat to make a total of 4 quesadillas. Serve with the salsa and sour cream, if using.

Makes 4 quesadillas

PER QUESADILLA: 450 calories, 26 g protein, 57 g carbohydrates, 11 g fat, 10 mg cholesterol, 840 mg sodium, 3 g dietary fiber

HEALTHY AND DELICIOUS SPINACH LASAGNA

- 2 cups fat-free ricotta cheese
- 1 package (10 ounces) frozen chopped spinach, thawed and squeezed dry
- 1 egg or ¼ cup liquid egg substitute
- 1 teaspoon dried basil
- ½ teaspoon Italian seasoning
- ½ teaspoon salt
- ¼ teaspoon ground black pepper
- 2 cups (8 ounces) part-skim mozzarella cheese
- 1 jar (28 ounces) spaghetti sauce
- 6 whole wheat lasagna noodles
- 1 cup water

Preheat the oven to 350°F.

In a medium bowl, combine the ricotta, spinach, egg or egg substitute, basil, Italian seasoning, salt, pepper, and 1 cup of the mozzarella.

Evenly spread one-third of the sauce in a 13" × 9" baking dish. Top with 3 lasagna noodles. Spread half of the cheese mixture over the noodles. Repeat. Top with the remaining sauce and the remaining 1 cup mozzarella. Add the water around the corners of the baking dish. Cover tightly with foil.

Bake for 1 hour and 15 minutes, or until hot and bubbly.

Makes 8 servings

PER SERVING: *310 calories, 19 g protein, 27 g carbohydrates, 15 g fat, 59 mg cholesterol, 913 mg sodium, 3 g dietary fiber*

FIVE-STAR VEGETABLE CHILI

1 teaspoon olive oil

1 onion, chopped

1 green bell pepper, chopped

2 cloves garlic, minced

1 jalapeño chile pepper, finely chopped (wear plastic gloves when handling), optional

1 tablespoon dried oregano

2 teaspoons chili powder

1 teaspoon ground cumin

1 can (28 ounces) no-salt-added diced tomatoes

1 can (15 ounces) no-salt-added tomato sauce

2 cups water

½ cup bulgur

2 cans (14–19 ounces each) beans, such as cannellini and/or kidney beans, rinsed and drained

Warm the oil in a Dutch oven over medium heat. Add the onion and bell pepper and cook, stirring occasionally, for 5 minutes, or until softened. Add the garlic, chile pepper, oregano, chili powder, and cumin and cook for 2 minutes.

Add the tomatoes (with juice), tomato sauce, and water. Increase the heat to medium-high and cook, stirring occasionally, for 5 minutes. Stir in the bulgur and beans. Reduce the heat to medium and cook for 15 minutes, or until thickened.

Makes 4 servings

PER SERVING: *341 calories, 14 g protein, 66 g carbohydrates, 3 g fat, 0 mg cholesterol, 430 mg sodium, 19 g dietary fiber*

HOPPIN' JOHN SALAD

2 slices turkey bacon

1 onion, chopped

2 cloves garlic, minced

3 cups fat-free chicken broth

½ cup wild rice, rinsed

1 teaspoon dried thyme

½ cup long-grain white rice

1 cup frozen black-eyed peas, thawed

1 rib celery, chopped

½ green bell pepper, chopped

1 small tomato, chopped

¼ cup chopped Italian parsley

2 tablespoons lemon juice

½ teaspoon hot-pepper sauce

¼ teaspoon ground black pepper

⅛ teaspoon salt

4 large beefsteak tomatoes

Cook the bacon in a medium saucepan over medium-high heat for 2 minutes, or until crisp. Remove from the pan and set aside until cool; crumble.

Add the onion and garlic to the same pan. Cook for 4 minutes, or until softened. Add the broth, wild rice, and thyme and bring to a boil. Cover, reduce the heat to low, and cook for 20 minutes.

Add the white rice. Cover and cook for 20 minutes, or until the rice is tender. Fluff the rice with a fork, loosely cover, and let cool completely.

Stir in the black-eyed peas, celery, bell pepper, chopped tomato, parsley, lemon juice, hot-pepper sauce, black pepper, salt, and crumbled bacon.

Slice the tops from the beefsteak tomatoes; carefully scoop out the insides and discard or reserve for another use. Divide the rice mixture among the tomatoes.

Makes 4 servings

PER SERVING: *299 calories, 16 g protein, 55 g carbohydrates, 2 g fat, 5 mg cholesterol, 360 mg sodium, 6 g dietary fiber*

BROWN RICE WITH PEPPERS AND ZUCCHINI

½ cup quick-cooking brown rice

1 packet or cube (1 teaspoon) beef or chicken bouillon

1 tablespoon olive oil

½ each red and yellow bell pepper, thinly sliced (¾ cup each)

½ zucchini, thinly sliced

1 tablespoon dried cilantro

½ teaspoon dried basil

½ teaspoon salt

Prepare the rice according to package directions, adding the bouillon to the water instead of salt.

Meanwhile, heat the oil in a large skillet over low heat. Add the bell peppers, zucchini, cilantro, basil, and salt. Increase the heat to medium and cook, stirring, for 3 minutes, or until crisp-tender. Serve the vegetables over the rice.

Makes 2 servings

PER SERVING: *210 calories, 4 g protein, 32 g carbohydrates, 8 g fat, 0 mg cholesterol, 1,020 mg sodium, 4 g dietary fiber*

FIERY FUSILLI

8 ounces fusilli

1 tablespoon olive oil

1 clove garlic, minced

2 banana chile peppers, finely chopped (wear plastic gloves when handling)

4 plum tomatoes, chopped

1 large roasted red pepper, chopped

2 tablespoons chopped Italian parsley

1 tablespoon chopped fresh sage

2 teaspoons chopped fresh oregano

⅛ teaspoon salt

1 can (14–19 ounces) chickpeas, rinsed and drained

½ cup fat-free chicken broth

¼ teaspoon crushed red-pepper flakes

Prepare the pasta according to the package directions. Drain and place in a serving bowl.

Meanwhile, heat the oil in a large nonstick skillet over medium-high heat. Add the garlic and chile peppers and cook for 2 minutes, or until the peppers are tender. Add the tomatoes, roasted pepper, parsley, sage, oregano, and salt and cook for 5 minutes, or until the tomatoes begin to release their juice. Add the chickpeas, broth, and red-pepper flakes and cook for 2 minutes. Pour the sauce over the pasta and toss to combine.

Makes 4 servings

PER SERVING: *389 calories, 15 g protein, 71 g carbohydrates, 6 g fat, 0 mg cholesterol, 420 mg sodium, 8 g dietary fiber*

HUMMUS SALAD

2 large carrots, chopped

2 tablespoons water

6 black olives, chopped

1 scallion, chopped

1 can (15 ounces) chickpeas

1 clove garlic

1 tablespoon grapeseed oil or other oil

Pinch of salt

Place the carrots and water in a microwaveable bowl. Cover with plastic wrap and microwave for 4 minutes, or until tender-crisp. Drain. Add the olives and scallion.

In a food processor or blender, combine the chickpeas, garlic, and oil until almost a smooth paste. Add to the carrot mixture and sprinkle with the salt. Stir to combine.

Makes 40 servings (1 tablespoon each)

PER TABLESPOON: *18 calories, 1 g protein, 3 g carbohydrates, 1 g fat, 0 mg cholesterol, 46 mg sodium, 1 g dietary fiber*

NOODLE-CRAB SALAD

1 pound tricolor rotini pasta

1 package (16 ounces) imitation crabmeat, flaked

1 rib celery, chopped

1 green bell pepper, chopped

½ small onion, chopped

½ cup reduced-fat mayonnaise

½ cup reduced-fat ranch salad dressing

1 teaspoon dried dillweed

Prepare the pasta according to package directions. Drain, rinse with cold water, and place in a serving bowl. Add the crabmeat, celery, pepper, and onion.

In a small bowl, combine the mayonnaise, salad dressing, and dill. Pour over the pasta mixture and toss to coat. Cover and refrigerate for at least 2 hours before serving.

Makes 8 servings

PER SERVING: *338 calories, 16 g protein, 58 g carbohydrate, 5 g fat, 31 mg cholesterol, 287 mg sodium, 2 g dietary fiber*

COUSCOUS SALAD

2 cups hot cooked couscous

2 roma tomatoes, cored, seeded, and chopped

¼ cup fresh basil leaves, snipped

1 clove garlic, minced

3 tablespoons balsamic vinegar

2 tablespoons olive oil

In a large serving bowl, combine the couscous, tomatoes, basil, garlic, vinegar, and oil. Toss to coat.

Makes 4 servings

PER SERVING: *163 calories, 3 g protein, 22 g carbohydrate, 7 g fat, 0 mg cholesterol, 10 mg sodium, 2 g dietary fiber*

EASY TASTY COTTAGE FRIES

3–4 large Idaho potatoes, sliced into half-dollar-size pieces

½ teaspoon seasoned pepper

½ teaspoon garlic salt

½ teaspoon ground paprika

Fat-free butter spray

Preheat the oven to 375°F.

Place the potatoes in a single layer on a baking sheet. Sprinkle with the pepper, garlic salt, and paprika. Coat with the butter spray.

Bake for 10 minutes, or until tender and lightly browned.

Makes 4 servings

PER SERVING: *102 calories, 4 g protein, 26 g carbohydrate, 0 g fat, 0 mg cholesterol, 120 mg sodium, 3 g dietary fiber*

QUICK SPINACH SAUTÉ

1–2 tablespoons olive oil

2 cloves garlic, crushed

1 cup sliced mushrooms

1 package (10 ounces) frozen chopped spinach, thawed and squeezed dry

½ cup grape tomatoes, halved

Place the oil and garlic in a cold skillet over medium heat for 2 minutes, or until the garlic is soft. Add the mushrooms and cook, stirring occasionally, for 5 minutes, or until the mushrooms release their liquid. Stir in the spinach and tomatoes and heat through.

Makes 4 servings

PER SERVING: *59 calories, 3 g protein, 5 g carbohydrate, 4 g fat, 0 mg cholesterol, 55 mg sodium, 3 g dietary fiber*

GOLD RUSH LEMON BARS

Crust

- 2 cups unbleached all-purpose flour
- ⅔ cup confectioners' sugar
- ½ cup butter or margarine, cut into small pieces

Filling

- 3 lemons
- 1½ cups sugar
- ¼ cup unbleached all-purpose flour
- 1 cup liquid egg substitute
- 2 tablespoons confectioners' sugar

To make the crust: Preheat the oven to 350°F. Coat a jelly-roll pan with cooking spray.

In a medium bowl, combine the flour and confectioners' sugar. Cut in the margarine or butter until the mixture resembles coarse meal. Press evenly into the bottom of the prepared pan. Bake for 10 minutes, or until lightly browned. Cool on a rack.

To make the filling: Grate the peel from 2 of the lemons into a medium bowl. Cut all the lemons in half and squeeze the juice into the bowl. Discard the lemons. Whisk in the sugar, flour, and egg substitute until smooth. Pour over the prepared crust. Bake for 18 minutes, or until the filling is set when lightly touched in the center and the edges are beginning to color. Cool on a rack. When completely cooled, sift the confectioners' sugar over the top.

Makes 36 bars

PER BAR: *98 calories, 2 g protein, 17 g carbohydrates, 3 g fat, 5 mg cholesterol, 10 mg sodium, 0 g dietary fiber*

CHOCOLATE CHEESECAKE

1½ cups chocolate cookie crumbs, finely crushed

2 tablespoons butter or margarine, melted

32 ounces low-fat cream cheese or soy cream cheese

1¼ cups sugar

2 eggs

1 egg white

6 ounces chocolate chips, melted and cooled slightly

1 cup soy sour cream

1 teaspoon vanilla extract

Preheat the oven to 325°F.

In a small bowl, combine the cookie crumbs and margarine. Press into the bottom of a 9" springform pan.

In a large bowl, with an electric mixer on medium speed, combine the cream cheese and sugar until well-blended. Add the eggs, one at a time, and egg white, beating well after each addition. Add the melted chocolate chips, sour cream, and vanilla extract and beat just until blended. Pour over the prepared crust.

Bake for 1 hour 25 minutes. Turn off the oven and leave in the oven for 1 hour. Remove to a rack to cool completely.

Makes 20 servings

PER SERVING: *269 calories, 7 g protein, 27 g carbohydrates, 15 g fat, 50 mg cholesterol, 250 mg sodium, 1 g dietary fiber*

APPLE CRISP

4 large Granny Smith apples, peeled and cut into ¼" slices

1 can (16 ounces) whole cranberries

1 tablespoon unbleached all-purpose flour

1 cup rolled oats (not quick-cooking)

2 tablespoons sugar

1 teaspoon ground cinnamon

¼ cup walnuts

4 tablespoons applesauce

Fat-free frozen whipped topping, thawed

Preheat the oven to 325°F. Coat an 8" × 8" baking dish with cooking spray.

Place the apples in the prepared baking dish. Combine the cranberries with the flour and toss with the apples.

In a food processor, combine the oats, sugar, cinnamon, and walnuts. Pulse, gradually adding the applesauce until the mixture starts to clump. Spoon over the cranberries.

Bake for 45 minutes, or until the apples are tender and the topping is lightly browned. Cover with foil, if necessary, to prevent browning too quickly. Serve with whipped topping.

Makes 6 servings

PER SERVING: *250 calories, 2 g protein, 53 g carbohydrates, 3 g fat, 0 mg cholesterol, 29 mg sodium, 4 g dietary fiber*

TIRAMISU

1 tablespoon + 1½ teaspoons instant espresso powder or 3 tablespoons instant coffee powder

½ cup + 1½ tablespoons hot water

32 ladyfingers, split

3 tablespoons seedless raspberry jam

3 egg whites, at room temperature

1 cup + 2 tablespoons sugar

3 tablespoons cold water

¼ teaspoon cream of tartar

4 ounces mascarpone cheese

4 ounces reduced-fat cream cheese, at room temperature

1 tablespoon semisweet chocolate shavings

Preheat the oven to 350°F.

In a small bowl, combine the espresso or coffee powder and ½ cup of the hot water. Brush the cut side of each ladyfinger with the mixture.

In another small bowl, combine the jam with the remaining 1½ tablespoons hot water to make a spreadable mixture. Brush the top side of each ladyfinger with a light coating of the mixture.

Bring about 2" water to a simmer in a large saucepan. In a medium heatproof bowl that will fit over the saucepan, combine the egg whites, sugar, cold water, and cream of tartar. Place the bowl over the saucepan. With an electric mixer on low speed, beat for 5 minutes. Increase the speed to high and beat for 4 minutes longer, or until very thick. Remove the bowl from the saucepan. Beat for 4 minutes, or until the mixture is very light and fluffy.

In a large bowl, combine the mascarpone and cream cheese. Using the same mixer, beat until creamy. Add 1 cup of the egg-white mixture and beat until smooth. Gradually fold in the remaining egg-white mixture.

Line the bottom and sides of a 2-quart serving bowl or a 9" × 9" baking dish with 16 of the ladyfingers, jam side up; top with one-fourth of the filling. Repeat 3 times to use all the ladyfingers and filling. Sprinkle with the chocolate.

Cover and refrigerate for at least 4 hours or up to 3 days before serving.

Makes 10 servings

PER SERVING: *299 calories, 6 g protein, 48 g carbohydrates, 10 g fat, 78 mg cholesterol, 330 mg sodium, 0 g dietary fiber*

CHOCOLATE MOUSSE

¾ cup 1% milk

1 tablespoon instant coffee powder

⅔ cup unsweetened cocoa powder

¼ cup packed light brown sugar

1 egg, lightly beaten

2 tablespoons coffee liqueur or strong brewed coffee

1 teaspoon unflavored gelatin

2 ounces bittersweet chocolate, coarsely chopped

1 tablespoon vanilla extract

4 egg whites

½ cup sugar

½ teaspoon cream of tartar

1 cup fat-free frozen whipped topping, thawed + additional for garnish (optional)

In a medium saucepan, combine the milk and coffee powder. Cook, stirring occasionally, over medium heat for 2 minutes, or until steaming. Whisk in the cocoa and brown sugar until smooth. Remove from the heat and slowly whisk in the egg. Reduce the heat to low and whisk constantly for 5 minutes, or until thickened. Remove from the heat.

Place the coffee liqueur or coffee in a cup. Sprinkle with the gelatin. Let stand for 1 minute to soften. Stir into the cocoa mixture until dissolved. Add the chocolate and vanilla extract and stir until the chocolate is melted. Place in a large bowl and set aside for 30 minutes, or until cooled to room temperature.

Bring 2" water to a simmer in a medium saucepan. In a large heatproof bowl that will fit over the saucepan, whisk together the egg whites, sugar, and cream of tartar. Set the bowl over the simmering water and gently whisk for 2 minutes, or until an instant-read thermometer registers 140°F (the mixture will be too hot to touch). Remove from the heat.

With an electric mixer on medium-high speed, beat for 5 minutes, or until cool. Fold the egg-white mixture into the chocolate mixture. Fold in the whipped topping. Divide among dessert glasses and refrigerate for at least 2 hours or up to 24 hours. Garnish with additional whipped topping, if using.

Makes 8 servings

PER SERVING: *176 calories, 5 g protein, 26 g carbohydrates, 5 g fat, 25 mg cholesterol, 55 mg sodium, 3 g dietary fiber*

NO-BAKE STRAWBERRY DESSERT

1 prepared angel food cake, cut into 1" cubes

2 packages (0.3 ounce each) sugar-free strawberry gelatin

2 cups boiling water

1 package (16–20 ounces) frozen unsweetened whole strawberries, thawed

2 cups 1% milk

1 package (1 ounce) sugar-free instant vanilla pudding mix

8 ounces reduced-fat frozen whipped topping, thawed

Place the cake cubes in a 13" × 9" baking dish.

In a medium bowl, combine the gelatin and water and stir to dissolve. Stir in the strawberries. Pour over the cake cubes in the pan and gently press cake down. Cover and refrigerate for 1 hour, or until set.

In another medium bowl, whisk together the milk and pudding mix for 2 minutes, or until slightly thickened. Spoon over the cake. Spread the whipped topping over the top. Cover and refrigerate until serving.

Makes 16 servings

PER SERVING: *145 calories, 4 g protein, 31 g carbohydrate, 0 g fat, 0 mg cholesterol, 240 mg sodium, 1 g dietary fiber*

APPENDIX

As discussed in Chapter 9, record keeping provides educational and motivational benefits that reinforce your training and reduce your chances of skipping workouts. Maintaining an accurate exercise log is perhaps the best way to monitor your training progress. And seeing more exercise repetitions and heavier exercise weight loads in successive training sessions is highly reinforcing and increases your incentive for regular workouts.

Training logs are also valuable tools for noting any problem areas, such as a lack of progress or regression in certain exercises. Such occurrences may indicate that you need to change an exercise or adjust your training protocol.

In addition to providing training accountability, each daily log sheet includes a section on your nutritional intake. Filling in your breakfast, lunch, dinner, and snack foods should be extremely helpful in monitoring and maintaining healthy eating patterns. For example, when you record your snacks on paper, you are more likely to choose high-nutrition snack foods, such as a yogurt smoothie, over high-calorie snack foods, like a chocolate milk shake.

Try to write down in your log your specific training goals for the day *before* your workout and to record your satisfaction rating *after* your workout. This is one of the best means for maintaining focus on your exercise performance as it relates to your training purpose.

Of course, the log is just a guide. Feel free to add your own categories of information to better accommodate your training interests and priorities.

GET STRONGER, FEEL YOUNGER DAILY TRAINING LOG

DAY _Monday_   DATE _11/12/07_   TIME _7:00 a.m._

TODAY'S GOALS: _Complete my strength exercise in 20 minutes, followed by a full 20 minutes of stationary cycling at level five._

Muscle: Strength Exercise   Yes ☑   No ☐

Satisfaction Rating   1   2   3   4   ⑤
                    (low)   (high)

HIGHLIGHTS AND COMMENTS: _Completed all of my strength exercises with good form in less than 20 minutes._

Cardio: Aerobic Exercise   Yes ☑   No ☐

Satisfaction Rating   1   2   3   ④   5
                    (low)   (high)

HIGHLIGHTS AND COMMENTS: _Did 15 minutes of stationary cycling at level five and 5 minutes at level four._

NUTRITION LOG

BREAKFAST _Raisin bagel, banana, orange juice_

LUNCH _Tuna sandwich, apple, V-8 juice_

DINNER _Chicken tenders, baked potato, sour cream, peas, tossed salad, whole wheat roll, tea, milk, apple crisp_

SNACKS _Yogurt, grapes, two cookies, milk_

EXERCISE LOG

EXERCISE	RESISTANCE	REPETITIONS	COMMENTS
1. Leg Extension	50	10	good set
2. Leg Curl	55	10	a little fast
3. Leg Press	120	12	125 next workout
4. Leg Extension	375	10	good set
5. Pulldown	45	11	poor last rep
6. Shoulder Press	30	9	felt hard
7. Biceps Curl	27.5	10	good set
8. Triceps Extension	25	11	good set
9. Lower Back Extension	60	12	62.5 next workout
10. Abdominal Curl	45	13	47.5 next workout
11.			
12.			
13.			
14.			
15.			
16.			
17.			
18.			

Fitness Reminder: *Unless you do regular strength training, you lose approximately ½ pound of muscle tissue each year (runners and aerobic exercisers included).*

GET STRONGER, FEEL YOUNGER DAILY TRAINING LOG

DAY _____ DATE _____ TIME _____

TODAY'S GOALS: _____

_____

_____

_____

Muscle: Strength Exercise   Yes ☐   No ☐

Satisfaction Rating   1   2   3   4   5
                      (low)   (high)

HIGHLIGHTS AND COMMENTS: _____

_____

_____

_____

Cardio: Aerobic Exercise   Yes ☐   No ☐

Satisfaction Rating   1   2   3   4   5
                      (low)   (high)

HIGHLIGHTS AND COMMENTS: _____

_____

_____

_____

NUTRITION LOG

BREAKFAST _____

_____

_____

LUNCH _____

_____

_____

DINNER _____

_____

_____

SNACKS _____

_____

_____

EXERCISE LOG

	EXERCISE	RESISTANCE	REPETITIONS	COMMENTS
1.				
2.				
3.				
4.				
5.				
6.				
7.				
8.				
9.				
10.				
11.				
12.				
13.				
14.				
15.				
16.				
17.				
18.				

Fitness Reminder: *Remodeling your muscle is by far the most effective means for achieving permanent fat loss.*

GET STRONGER, FEEL YOUNGER DAILY TRAINING LOG

DAY _____ DATE _____ TIME _____

TODAY'S GOALS:_____

_____

_____

_____

Muscle: Strength Exercise   Yes ☐   No ☐

Satisfaction Rating   1   2   3   4   5
                     (low)   (high)

HIGHLIGHTS AND COMMENTS: _____

_____

_____

_____

Cardio: Aerobic Exercise   Yes ☐   No ☐

Satisfaction Rating   1   2   3   4   5
                     (low)   (high)

HIGHLIGHTS AND COMMENTS: _____

_____

_____

_____

NUTRITION LOG

BREAKFAST_____

_____

_____

LUNCH _____

_____

_____

DINNER_____

_____

_____

SNACKS_____

_____

_____

EXERCISE LOG

	EXERCISE	RESISTANCE	REPETITIONS	COMMENTS
1.				
2.				
3.				
4.				
5.				
6.				
7.				
8.				
9.				
10.				
11.				
12.				
13.				
14.				
15.				
16.				
17.				
18.				

Fitness Reminder: *A slower metabolism is the primary cause of fat gain.*

GET STRONGER, FEEL YOUNGER DAILY TRAINING LOG

DAY _____ DATE _____ TIME _____

TODAY'S GOALS: _____

_____

_____

_____

Muscle: Strength Exercise   Yes ☐   No ☐

Satisfaction Rating   1   2   3   4   5
                        (low)   (high)

HIGHLIGHTS AND COMMENTS: _____

_____

_____

_____

Cardio: Aerobic Exercise   Yes ☐   No ☐

Satisfaction Rating   1   2   3   4   5
                        (low)   (high)

HIGHLIGHTS AND COMMENTS: _____

_____

_____

_____

NUTRITION LOG

BREAKFAST _____

_____

_____

LUNCH _____

_____

_____

DINNER _____

_____

_____

SNACKS _____

_____

_____

EXERCISE LOG

	EXERCISE	RESISTANCE	REPETITIONS	COMMENTS
1.				
2.				
3.				
4.				
5.				
6.				
7.				
8.				
9.				
10.				
11.				
12.				
13.				
14.				
15.				
16.				
17.				
18.				

Fitness Reminder: *By sensible training, we mean two or three training sessions a week for just 20 to 30 minutes per session.*

GET STRONGER, FEEL YOUNGER DAILY TRAINING LOG

DAY _____ DATE _____ TIME _____

TODAY'S GOALS:_____

_____

_____

_____

Muscle: Strength Exercise   Yes ☐   No ☐

Satisfaction Rating   1   2   3   4   5
                          (low)   (high)

HIGHLIGHTS AND COMMENTS: _____

_____

_____

_____

Cardio: Aerobic Exercise   Yes ☐   No ☐

Satisfaction Rating   1   2   3   4   5
                          (low)   (high)

HIGHLIGHTS AND COMMENTS: _____

_____

_____

_____

NUTRITION LOG

BREAKFAST_____

_____

LUNCH _____

_____

DINNER_____

_____

SNACKS_____

_____

EXERCISE LOG

	EXERCISE	RESISTANCE	REPETITIONS	COMMENTS
1.				
2.				
3.				
4.				
5.				
6.				
7.				
8.				
9.				
10.				
11.				
12.				
13.				
14.				
15.				
16.				
17.				
18.				

Fitness Reminder: *Typical diet plans result in more muscle loss and metabolic rate reduction, because approximately 25 percent of the weight loss is actually muscle tissue.*

GET STRONGER, FEEL YOUNGER DAILY TRAINING LOG

DAY _____ DATE _____ TIME _____

TODAY'S GOALS:_____
_____
_____
_____

Muscle: Strength Exercise   Yes ☐   No ☐

Satisfaction Rating   1   2   3   4   5
                      (low)   (high)

HIGHLIGHTS AND COMMENTS: _____
_____
_____
_____

Cardio: Aerobic Exercise   Yes ☐   No ☐

Satisfaction Rating   1   2   3   4   5
                      (low)   (high)

HIGHLIGHTS AND COMMENTS: _____
_____
_____
_____

NUTRITION LOG

BREAKFAST_____
_____
_____

LUNCH _____
_____
_____

DINNER_____
_____
_____

SNACKS_____
_____
_____

EXERCISE LOG

	EXERCISE	RESISTANCE	REPETITIONS	COMMENTS
1.				
2.				
3.				
4.				
5.				
6.				
7.				
8.				
9.				
10.				
11.				
12.				
13.				
14.				
15.				
16.				
17.				
18.				

Fitness Reminder: *Reduced-calorie diets almost always result in decreased energy.*

GET STRONGER, FEEL YOUNGER DAILY TRAINING LOG

DAY _____ DATE _____ TIME _____

TODAY'S GOALS:_____

_____

_____

_____

Muscle: Strength Exercise   Yes ☐   No ☐

Satisfaction Rating   1   2   3   4   5
                    (low)   (high)

HIGHLIGHTS AND COMMENTS: _____

_____

_____

_____

Cardio: Aerobic Exercise   Yes ☐   No ☐

Satisfaction Rating   1   2   3   4   5
                    (low)   (high)

HIGHLIGHTS AND COMMENTS: _____

_____

_____

_____

NUTRITION LOG

BREAKFAST_____

_____

_____

LUNCH _____

_____

_____

DINNER_____

_____

_____

SNACKS _____

_____

_____

EXERCISE LOG

EXERCISE	RESISTANCE	REPETITIONS	COMMENTS
1.			
2.			
3.			
4.			
5.			
6.			
7.			
8.			
9.			
10.			
11.			
12.			
13.			
14.			
15.			
16.			
17.			
18.			

Fitness Reminder: *Unlike dieting, strength training builds muscle tissue and increases your resting metabolic rate.*

GET STRONGER, FEEL YOUNGER DAILY TRAINING LOG

DAY _____ DATE _____ TIME _____

TODAY'S GOALS:_____

_____

_____

_____

Muscle: Strength Exercise   Yes ☐   No ☐

Satisfaction Rating   1   2   3   4   5
                      (low)   (high)

HIGHLIGHTS AND COMMENTS: _____

_____

_____

_____

Cardio: Aerobic Exercise   Yes ☐   No ☐

Satisfaction Rating   1   2   3   4   5
                      (low)   (high)

HIGHLIGHTS AND COMMENTS: _____

_____

_____

_____

NUTRITION LOG

BREAKFAST_____

_____

_____

LUNCH _____

_____

_____

DINNER_____

_____

_____

SNACKS_____

_____

_____

EXERCISE LOG

	EXERCISE	RESISTANCE	REPETITIONS	COMMENTS
1.				
2.				
3.				
4.				
5.				
6.				
7.				
8.				
9.				
10.				
11.				
12.				
13.				
14.				
15.				
16.				
17.				
18.				

Fitness Reminder: *Muscle-building exercise actually has a double effect on energy utilization in that it causes calories to burn both during and after the strength-training workout.*

INDEX

Boldface page references indicate photographs. <u>Underscored</u> references indicate boxed text or charts.